LOSE YOUR

INCHES

WITHOUT

LOSING YOUR

MIND!

LOSE YOUR INCHES WITHOUT LOSING YOUR MIND!

10 SIMPLE WEEKS
to a Slimmer Waistline and a Healthier You

Justine SanFilippo, MS, CHC

RIVER GROVE
BOOKS

This book is intended as a reference volume only, not as a medical manual. The information given here is designed to help you make informed decisions about your health. It is not intended as a substitute for any treatment that may have been prescribed by your doctor. If you suspect that you have a medical problem, you should seek competent medical help. You should not begin a new health regimen without first consulting a medical professional.

Published by River Grove Books
Austin, TX
www.rivergrovebooks.com

Distributed by River Grove Books

For ordering information or special discounts for bulk purchases, please contact River Grove Books at PO Box 91869, Austin, TX 78709, 512.891.6100.

Design and composition by Greenleaf Book Group
Cover design by Debbie Berne and Greenleaf Book Group
Cover: brunette illustration © Kakigori Studio. Used under license from Shutterstock.com

Cataloging-in-Publication data

SanFilippo, Justine.

   Lose your inches without losing your mind! : 10 simple weeks to a slimmer waistline and a healthier you / Justine SanFilippo, MS, CHC.—First edition.

   pages : illustrations ; cm

   Issued also as an ebook.

   Includes bibliographical references.

   ISBN: 978-1-938416-91-0

   1. Weight loss. 2. Weight loss—Psychological aspects. 3. Nutrition. 4. Physical fitness. 5. Health. I. Title.

RM222.2 .S26 2014

613.25   2014935724

First Edition

Other Editions:
eBook ISBN: 978-1-938416-91-0

I would like to dedicate this book to my family—
particularly my mom Jennifer and my dad George.

My mother has always been a big influence in my life regarding the love
of health. Mom, thank you for being a great mother and friend, for your
unconditional support, and for being an inspiration for me to follow my path.
Dad, thank you for giving me the advice, "Do what you love because then
you'll never work a day in your life." I truly appreciate your patience, guidance,
and unwavering support throughout my journey.

CONTENTS

AUTHOR'S NOTE

Lose Your Inches without Losing Your Mind! will tell you my story and the stories of my clients—all the crazy things I've tried to lose those inches and how I finally figured out a way to keep them off . . . for good!

You may have already lost your mind, which is why you picked up this book. You may just be starting to lose your mind and would like to get it back before you fall off the rocker completely. You may have seen others lose their minds with all sorts of crazy diets, so the mere thought of attempting one yourself is almost too much to handle.

Whatever your state of mind-loss is right now, my goal is to show you what worked for me and how it can work for you, too. I want to save you the heartache, confusion, and mental exhaustion of figuring out how to shrink your waistline. If you want to lose inches and keep your sanity, then this is the book for you.

Follow me! Let's start losing your inches *without* losing your mind!

INTRODUCTION
Breaking Up with Your Scale

> **How to *Not* Lose Your Mind: Introductory Lesson**
>
> Breaking up with your scale is like breaking off any relationship. At first you may feel weird not having it in your daily life, but then it gets easier, day by day. Remember that boyfriend or girlfriend you thought you couldn't live without—but you don't give a second thought about them now? The same thing will happen when you break up with your scale. Your mood and mind will stay sane!

I know. That cold piece of metal is sitting on the bathroom floor, waiting for you faithfully each morning to step on it. You've had a relationship with it for so long that it seems like an eternity. But for some reason, you feel that your scale is not always fair to you. It doesn't always give you what you want out of the relationship.

One of two things will happen after you weigh yourself during this morning ritual: You will either be very excited or you will feel very depressed for the whole day. Many of us let that little scale actually determine what kind of day we're going to have and what our mood is going to be. We let the scale influence everything: from how we look at ourselves in the mirror to how we feel around our significant other. We even let this piece of metal determine how we will eat that day.

Why do we let this inanimate object have such a hold over us? Why do we put ourselves through this torture every morning? Well, first of all, it's a habit, and like most habits, we simply may not know how to break it. Let's try logic first.

For example, if you go to bed at one weight and wake up the next morning 2 pounds heavier, you need to know that it is *literally impossible* to gain 2 pounds overnight in actual weight—water weight, maybe, but not actual weight. You would have had to consume something like 7,000 extra calories (3,500 × 2) the day before with no activity whatsoever. One pound = 3,500 calories. I don't think it is possible to eat that much even on Thanksgiving! So, when you wake up in the morning and are up or down by a few pounds, it's usually just water weight. Did you drink alcohol the night before? Did you eat anything salty? Did you eat sugar? Did you drink just coffee and diet soda yesterday and forget to drink water? So many things make our weight fluctuate.

How did that logical reasoning work for you? Feeling a little more sane? I know: It's tough using logic against an obsession. Some of you even (gasp!) weigh yourselves several times a day. Save yourself the heartache, please! Your weight can sometimes vary up to 7 pounds in one day from morning to evening, depending on what you are eating, what you are drinking, and what your activity level is. These variations that occur naturally throughout the day cannot determine your actual weight.

Like many of you, I have been on a zillion diets in my lifetime. It took me many years to figure out how to reach my ideal size without that scale. I used to be one of those people who checked my weight several times a day. If I can make progress, so can you! Now I only weigh myself when I go to the doctor's office or a few times a month when I dig out my scale from the back of my closet. Your progress toward achieving your ideal size can be greatly affected by your mood, so let's make sure you're in a good mood every day. Here are the four steps to breaking up with your scale:

Step 1: Reduce Your Visits. The first step to breaking up with your scale is to only visit it once a week (I recommend that eventually you weigh yourself less often than that—more like once a month). Visit your scale on the same morning of the same day each week, after you've gone to the bathroom; for example, every Monday. Until that day comes along, the scale needs to be hidden.

Step 2: Hide It. I don't care where you put it—somewhere inconvenient is ideal. Try the garage, the attic, the back of your closet, or the bottom of the dirty laundry bin. When you are only weighing yourself once a week or less, you can get a better idea of how you are progressing toward reaching your goals. Even on my favorite show, *The Biggest Loser*, the contestants only weigh themselves once a week.

Step 3: Appreciate What You See. When you wake up each day, instead of weighing yourself, look at your body in the mirror. How do you feel? What do you appreciate about what you see? How do your *pants fit* that day? Appreciating how you look *today* and knowing you are on the right path makes those inches come off faster.

Step 4: Pick a Favorite Pair of Pants. I believe that the best indication of how inch-loss progress is going is by how your pants fit. Choose a pair of pants that don't shrink or stretch and try them on. That single pair of pants can tell you much more than a scale can. I have one pair of jeans that don't shrink or stretch, and they are the sole indicator I use to determine if I need to increase my exercise or if I'm right where I need to be.

Voila! Breaking up with your scale is as easy as steps 1, 2, 3, and 4.

WEEK 1

Baby Goals and Baby Steps

> **How to *Not* Lose Your Mind: Lesson for Week 1**
>
> Breaking goals down into "baby steps" makes them feel much easier to achieve and more attainable. Why overwhelm yourself for no reason? Baby steps are the key to everything. Relax your mind and learn like a baby—one step at a time!

As we read in the last section, the scale can fluctuate quite a bit during a two-day span or even during the same day from morning to evening. This can be very frustrating. Many factors determine what the scale communicates to you in the morning. When you step on the scale, it measures fat, muscle, water, food, the glass of orange juice or coffee you just drank, and the salt/water retention from last night's dinner. The scale can go up by several pounds one day, yet your pants—what we might call the "eye test"—may indicate no change.

LEARNING HOW TO MEASURE

Measuring by how your pants fit—now, that's sanity! Using inches as a measuring tool makes sense because inches indicate the actual shape of the body. Have you ever seen a skinny-fat person? Someone who has no muscle tone, whose arms and stomach just sort of sag on his or her frame? Often this is what happens when people try to lose weight just for weight's sake. You can actually lose a lot of muscle if you lose weight too quickly.

This is also what happens with yo-yo dieting. Those who are up, down, then back up again lose weight in a short period of time, but what they have actually lost is mostly water and muscle. Then they eat like normal people, and the weight piles on as fast as possible. Why? Because these individuals have lost a lot of muscle with all the dieting, resulting in their metabolism slowing down. Muscle burns about 6 calories per pound while at rest, while fat only burns 2 calories per pound.[1] So, if you are on a starvation diet, for example, and lose 10 pounds of muscle, you're actually burning 60 fewer calories per day. That may not sound like a lot, but to put it in perspective, in one year you would burn 21,900 fewer calories, which would equal sizeble weight gain over the course of the year. Your metabolism suffers, and besides doing damage to your overall state of health, you actually have no chance of keeping those pounds off in the long run.

Now get this: Inches are more important than weight, not only for your sanity, but also for your actual health. There are several scientific measurements for body composition: Body Mass Index (BMI), Waist-to-Hip Ratio (WHR), waist circumference, and body fat percentage. We are going to focus on BMI and waist circumference.

BMI is a good example of a measurement that simply uses weight in relationship to a person's height. However, the issue with BMI is that a person who is extremely fit and very muscular can be classified as "overweight" or even "obese," even with a low body fat percentage. For example, I once knew a girl who lost 135 pounds. It was amazing how she transformed her body, and she became extremely toned and muscular. She was 5'2", weighed 139 pounds, and wore a size 2. Using a BMI chart, she would technically be overweight. Believe me, she was definitely not overweight! She was in amazing condition, and you could see every muscle.

Waist circumference is a much better indicator of a person's overall health. This measurement has a direct correlation to a person's risk for heart disease, which is one of the main causes of death in the United States. Most men tend to carry weight in their bellies, which

---

1   Z. Wang, Z. Ying, A. Bosy-Westphal, J. Zhang, B. Schautz, W. Later, S. B. Heymsfield, and M. J. Muller, "Specific Metabolic Rates of Major Organs and Tissues across Adulthood: Evaluation by Mechanistic Model of Resting Energy Expenditure," *American Journal of Clinical Nutrition* 92, no. 6 (December 2010):1369–77, doi:10.3945/ajcn.2010.29885. Available at http://www.ncbi .nlm.nih.gov/pubmed/20962155.

they affectionately call their "beer gut" or "love handles." This is called *android obesity*. Men need to keep their waistline less than 40 inches, otherwise they are at risk for several health issues. Many studies have shown that those with android obesity are at a greater risk for insulin resistance, elevated insulin levels, type 2 diabetes, hypertension, high blood pressure, high cholesterol and triglyceride levels, stroke, metabolic syndrome, and ultimately an early death.

Women tend to carry more weight in their thighs and hips, which is called *gynoid obesity*. Women need to keep their waistlines less than 35 inches to be considered healthy. Extra weight in the waistline can lead to an increased risk for hypertension, type 2 diabetes, metabolic syndrome, high cholesterol, and high triglyceride levels.[2]

Again, healthy waist measurements for men and women are:

* Men < 40 inches
* Women < 35 inches

Which system of measurement sounds more accurate and important to you? I'm telling you, it's the inches!

This book is designed for you to follow a 10-week program, week-by-week, so that I can walk you through how to *Lose Your Inches without Losing Your Mind!* Some of you will read the whole book in one sitting, which is fine, but if you try to implement all the steps at once, it will be too overwhelming and not as effective. I highly encourage you to only read one chapter per week and follow the directions. Together, we will create baby goals for you to follow each week. You will also take your measurements at the beginning of each week. By the end of the book, you will have built a foundation of healthy habits to last you throughout your life and will be able to compare your overall inches from Week 1 to Week 10.

Our first action step is to take actual measurements of your body. Get a $2 soft measuring tape at any grocery or convenience store and measure different areas of the body: waist, hips, lower abdomen,

2   Robert D. Lee and David C. Neiman, *Nutritional Assessment,* 5th ed. (New York: McGraw-Hill, 2010), 179.

thighs, chest, arms, and calves. Take these measurements every week and write them down in the space provided in this book. Then, add them together to get one total. Comparing your total inches every week is going to be your new way to measure your progress. Your disappearing inches are a much greater indicator of how things are going toward achieving your ideal size. You can also view my website at www.happyhealthypeople.com to view a FREE video of how to take your measurements.

Starting Measurements

_____ Waist (1 in. above belly button)

_____ Hips (widest part, around glutes)

_____ Lower abdomen (2 in. below belly button)

_____ Right thigh (put right hand flat against leg and measure under the thumb area)

_____ Left thigh (put left hand flat against leg and measure under the thumb area)

_____ Chest (measure around widest part)

_____ Right arm (measure around bicep area)

_____ Left arm (measure around bicep area)

_____ Right calf (measure around widest part)

_____ Left calf (measure around widest part)

_____ BEGINNING INCHES TOTAL

Before we move on to the next section, I want to mention (and refute) the biggest misconception about fat vs. muscle. That misconception goes something like this: "Everyone has heard that muscle weighs more than fat . . ." A pound is a pound is a pound, so technically muscle doesn't "weigh more" than fat. However, muscle *is* more dense than fat, and I know we all want to be more dense and less round. I remember when I owned a gym, we actually had two visuals—one was a soft, blubbery, squishy, yellow piece of "fat" that weighed 1 pound. It was about the size of a small football. The other visual was a 1-pound piece of "muscle" that was small, dense, red, and about the size of a baseball. They both weighed exactly 1 pound, but which would you choose? To be the size of a football or the size of a baseball? Exactly.

Another misconception is that if you start to work out, you will bulk up. This is an understandable but confused line of thinking. Yes, I will be getting you to work out and gain muscle, but does that mean you will bulk up like a professional bodybuilder? Not likely. Even if your goal is to gain a lot of muscle, reaching that goal will depend on your training efforts and mostly on the amount that you eat. Typically, professional bodybuilders eat much more than you think! Many bodybuilders also do some interesting things with supplements, and some even use testosterone or steroids. So, we're not going to go there.

Instead, it has been my experience that when clients first start to work out, they will shrink in the exact opposite areas where they first gained size. For example, if a woman gained inches in her thighs first, then glutes (glutes are short for the *gluteus maximus*, or the rear end), stomach, arms, and chest, typically she'll lose inches in this order: chest, arms, stomach, glutes, and thighs. There is absolutely *no* scientific proof of this; it's just what I've observed after working with hundreds of clients. Women in general tend to lose size in their chest first because, well, breasts are mostly just fat. Sorry ladies, but it's true!

If you are working out and lifting weights, it is quite possible that your scale will not change at all, or maybe it will only change by a few pounds. But your body measurements will be different. *Those inches will change!* I know from personal experience that my scale says the same thing that it has for years and years, but I am a size smaller than

I was a few years ago. Why? Because muscle is more dense than fat, as we just learned.

Losing inches is more important than losing weight because it reflects your actual state of improved health. It is also important because the more inches you lose, the more muscle you have gained. The more muscle you gain, the *leaner* and more *toned* you look, which is the entire goal, right? Right!

SETTING BABY GOALS AND TAKING BABY STEPS

When people look at me today, I'm sure some of them think, "Look at that girl. How is it that she eats whatever she wants and stays thin?" The answer: Every single day I make choices about food, exercise, and nutrition, just like you. Throughout this book you will read just how far from perfect I am, as we all are. It is important to understand that all of us face different challenges and decisions every day. None of us are perfect. Once you understand that being "perfect" is not an ideal goal, you are ready to make better, healthier choices that work for you.

Baby steps are about making small decisions each day; about carefully considering questions such as "What will I eat?" "Will I exercise today?" and "What is my body telling me?" In the long haul, these small choices will lead to big results. Baby steps will help you reach your goals, which we will break down into attainable objectives, or baby goals.

Everyone wants to lose 20 pounds in a day, but that's impossible. If it were possible, the United States would be the skinniest country in the world and not the heaviest. Most of us willingly jump on each new diet bandwagon or try the newest weight-loss pill just to see if we've found the miracle quick-fix. But do you know anyone who has ever done a fad diet and successfully kept the weight off permanently? I don't.

What happens when you begin a diet program? The first week is fantastic. The pounds seem to melt off, right? In reality, this weight loss is mostly water weight with some muscle, as we explored in the previous section. Once you start to eat a little cleaner or exercise, your body naturally starts to detox, which includes ridding itself of excess water. The body thinks you are wising up, so it starts to purge itself of all the toxins.

If you've ever watched *The Biggest Loser*—my favorite show in the world—you'll notice that the more contestants weigh in the beginning, the more they lose the first week. The heavier they are, the quicker they'll drop pounds. In your first week, you may lose anywhere from 1 to 10 pounds, but only a few of those pounds are actual fat weight.

What happens next—raise your hands if you've been there—is that after this first magnificent week or two, your results become increasingly less dramatic. Then your weight-loss plan goes completely off the rails, and you give up due to the frustration of not seeing results.

To get your weight-loss plan back on track, you need to set realistic baby goals rather than "I want to lose 20 pounds, stat." The solution? Start small. A good first baby goal could be as simple as "I want to eat breakfast every day," or "I want to get an hour more of sleep each night," or "I want to walk for 30 minutes, three times a week."

Throughout this book, I will be asking you to choose three baby goals per week. The idea is that you can add three new baby goals each week, once you have the old ones down pat. It's kind of like juggling: getting a few more balls in the air at a time, but you can do it!

For example, let's say this week I've decided my baby goal is just to walk 30 minutes, three days a week. This would be a good goal for someone who hasn't exercised in years and wants to ease back into it. Keep in mind that if need be, you can do 15 minutes in the morning and 15 minutes in the evening—whatever works for you to get your body moving.

What will end up happening is that you will feel *so good* at the end of the week when you go walking that you will naturally want to keep that baby goal for the following week! Not only that, but you will also have a sense of accomplishment that you *achieved your goal*, which in itself can be highly motivating. Let's say that your baby goal is "to not have that candy bar snack at 3:00 p.m., and to eat an apple instead." Or, your baby goal is "to drink one extra glass of water each day." Again, you will find that such small changes are easy to keep, so you will naturally want to keep it up week by week, achieving a domino effect.

When I coach clients, I have found that baby goals are the key to their success, just as small steps will be the key to your success. Here are thirty examples of baby goals you can use throughout this book as the weeks progress. Since you will be focusing on three goals per week, feel free to reference this list as we go along to get ideas for your baby goals. I will also have sample goals at the end of each chapter to guide you.

Sample Baby Goals

I will eat breakfast within 45 minutes of waking up.

I will walk for 30 minutes, three times a week.

I will eat a healthy snack between breakfast and lunch.

I will eat a healthy snack between lunch and dinner.

I will eat a healthier snack at 3:00 p.m., instead of a candy bar.

I will set a timer on my cell phone/watch/kitchen timer to remind myself to eat every three hours.

I will never go more than three hours without eating.

I will drink decaf coffee or tea instead of caffeinated.

I will cut all artificial sweeteners out of my diet and will try natural sweeteners instead, such as stevia or raw honey.

I will not weigh myself every day.

I will go to bed earlier and get one more hour of sleep per night.

I will pay attention to my portions when going out to eat.

I will look up the nutritional information of a restaurant's menu before dining out.

I will pay attention to my portions when eating at home.

I will start to read the labels on packages to learn about the ingredients.

I will look up the calories of my favorite foods online so I know what the heck I am eating.

I will pack my lunch three times a week.

I will have healthy snacks with me/in my purse/in my car/at my desk at all times.

I will carry a water bottle with me everywhere.

I will make sure I drink three to four bottles of water or eight to ten glasses of water per day.

I will limit my alcohol consumption to once a week or less.

I will try a new leafy green.

I will shop for organic produce.

I will try the local farmer's market.

I will eat more protein with each meal.

I will turn off the TV and computer one hour before bedtime.

I will try a new fruit.

I will walk into a gym and inquire about their programs.

I will contact a personal trainer and set up a free session with him or her.

I will clean my pantry and fridge of all the junk food that tempts me every single day.

As you can see, this list can truly go on and on. Make your goals easy and attainable. After all, they'll eventually build on top of each other. Pick three baby goals each week and focus on just those objectives.

Put your goals where you can easily see them first thing in the morning. I like to put mine on my bathroom mirror. You can also place them on the refrigerator, on your cell phone, or on your computer. When you are reminded each day of what you have set out to do, you will feel proud of yourself when you achieve your goals.

You will be surprised by how these baby goals will naturally lead to loftier ambitions. When you start with success instead of failure, you'll be so proud of yourself that you will want to set even more goals!

If I were just beginning this program, my three baby goals for my first week might be:

1. I will have healthy snacks on me at all times.
2. I will eat breakfast.
3. I will drink more water and carry a water bottle with me.

So what are your three baby goals for Week 1? What are three easy things you can focus on for *this* week? Feel free to reference the previous list of sample baby goals to get some ideas.

My three baby goals for this week are:

1. _____

   _____

2. _____

   _____

3. _____

   _____

WEEK 2

Learn How to Count

How to *Not* Lose Your Mind: Lesson for Week 2

Counting is one of the most important things we learned in grade school. Applying counting to your "Lose Your Inches" plan will help those inches fall off faster and easier so you won't get frustrated and go crazy. You'll be able to see exactly what is going on and why your pants are still tight or why they are getting looser. The difference between counting now and counting in grade school is that here you can estimate and you won't get a grade. I'll give you an "A" for effort *and* a gold star!

I know what you're thinking right now: "I don't want to count calories! Isn't there an easier way?"

Well . . . no, there's not. If you're serious about losing your inches, you have to count—at first. The good news is that you can learn to estimate calories as you go along until it becomes second nature. *Estimate*, not be exact. The more you know, the more you can apply this knowledge to reach your goals quicker. Remember—knowledge is power!

LEARNING HOW TO COUNT

The quickest way to start learning how to count is to look up the calories of your favorite foods. There are plenty of websites available for reference, such as the U. S. Department of Agriculture's website (www.nutrition.gov), which gives great, comprehensive nutritional information. You can also go to the USDA National Nutrient Database (http://ndb.nal.usda.gov). Type in any food and it will show you the calorie and nutrition content of that food. I also like www.nutritiondata.self.com and www.calorieking.com. Both of these websites are very easy to navigate, so you may want to try them first. To make it easier, there are also many free apps you can download to your cell phone that make it easy to not only discover the calories in a food but also to record those calories. One of my favorite apps is MyFitnessPal. Don't we all pretty much have a fancy cell phone these days? Well, in case you don't, they also have a website: www.myfitnesspal.com. There is also a chart in appendix I at the back of this book that lists common healthy foods and their calories.

The fact is that most people eat the same basic foods regularly. Foods that I eat often are eggs, oatmeal, high-fiber cereal, meat, poultry, fish, seafood, protein shakes and bars, nuts, fruit, vegetables, and chocolate (well, just a little). When I first started counting calories, I looked up how many calories were in each item, which helped me learn what a portion is. Then I kept track of my daily food and beverage intake on a little notepad I carried around in my purse. I did this routine for a while until it became second nature and I knew exactly what I was eating.

Later we'll discuss in more detail how to navigate portion sizes, but first I want you to use the next page to make a list of your favorite foods, and then go look up the calories in each food item. Again, refer to appendix I on page 157 for some basic foods and their calorie content if you don't have a cell phone or a computer. Try to list at least your top twenty favorite foods and beverages. Realistically, this list of twenty foods probably entails about 80 percent of what you normally consume each week. List the foods you regularly eat for each meal, and don't forget those desserts and between-meal snacks. Also, list beverages you normally consume, including alcohol, and of course that super-duper chocolate double latte cappuccino topped with whipped cream, sprinkles, and a maraschino cherry . . .

MY TOP 20 FAVORITE FOODS AND BEVERAGES

Food/Beverage	Calories
1.	
2.	
3.	
4.	
5.	
6.	
7.	
8.	
9.	
10.	
11.	
12.	
13.	
14.	
15.	
16.	
17.	
18.	
19.	
20.	

SO, HOW MANY CALORIES SHOULD I EAT?

It is important to know how many calories you should eat in order to reach your goals quickly. There's nothing worse than doing everything right, knowing the caloric value of everything you eat, writing down what you eat in your food log, exercising, drinking water, and having your waistline stay exactly the same after months of work. I know; I've done this! Before I understood what a calorie was, I was on a high-protein/low-carb diet and accidentally eating about 4,000 calories a day. I worked out almost every day, hired a personal trainer, and stuck to that diet perfectly. The only thing was, I never learned how many calories I should be eating.

So, let me save you a little frustration here and guide you in the right direction. There are a million formulas out there to calculate how much you should be eating, based on your lifestyle, activity, and goals. I'm going to give you the simplest scientific formula there is. It's called the Harris-Benedict equation, and it goes like this . . .

First, you calculate your BMR, which is your basal metabolic rate. This is how many calories your body needs to survive if you were just lying in bed all day and never moved. After all—your breathing, your heart beating, and your brain functioning all burn calories. For adults, the calculation is

Women:

655 + (4.35 × weight in pounds) + (4.7 × height in inches)
− (4.7 × age in years)

Men:

66 + (6.23 × weight in pounds) + (12.7 × height in inches)
− (6.8 × age in years)

Next, you need to factor in your *activity level*. This will give you your Active Metabolic Rate (AMR), which is the amount of calories you typically burn each day.

Sedentary = BMR × 1.2

(little or no exercise, desk job)

Lightly active = BMR × 1.375

(light exercise/sports, 1–3 days/wk)

Moderately active = BMR × 1.55

(moderate exercise/sports, 3–5 days/wk)

Very active = BMR × 1.725

(hard exercise/sports 6–7 days/wk)

Extremely active = BMR × 1.9

(hard daily exercise/sports & physical job or 2x day training, i.e., marathon runner, etc.)

When you multiply your BMR times your activity level, what is that number? This magic number gives you the number of calories you need to consume in a day to *maintain* your current weight.

BMR × ACTIVITY = NUMBER OF CALORIES NEEDED TO MAINTAIN CURRENT WEIGHT AND SIZE

Now, if you want to *lose inches*, you need to take in less than this number. Ideally, subtract 250 calories from this number to figure out how many you should consume a day. Then, you want to *burn* another 250 calories per day doing exercise. That way, you will create a total deficit of about 500 calories a day, which means you will lose inches and about 1 to 2 pounds per week. One pound is equal to 3,500 calories. You do want to make sure, however, to never go lower than your original BMR number through food or exercise. If you do, your body will then go into starvation mode, you won't lose any weight or inches, and you'll just get frustrated.

Losing 1 to 2 pounds per week is a safe, healthy way to lose inches and weight. You want to lose those inches and pounds at a slow rate so they don't come back! Unwanted weight didn't magically appear over-night, nor will it disappear overnight. As we will see in later weeks, you never want to create your caloric deficit based on lowering your food intake alone. It should be both caloric intake *and* exercise to produce optimal results.

Here is a sample of a female who is forty years old, weighs 160 pounds, and is 5'5". She works out three times per week and has a desk job. She would do the following calculation:

$$655 + (4.35 \times 160 \text{ lbs.}) + (4.7 \times 65 \text{ in.}) - (4.7 \times 40 \text{ years old}) = ????$$
$$655 + 696 + 305.5 - 188 = 1,468.5 \text{ calories/day BMR}$$

So, this woman burns 1,468.5 calories per day *if she lies in bed all day and never moves.* Basically, if she eats less than that, her body will go into starvation mode.

Now, let's calculate what she burns each day with her activity.

> 1,468.5 × 1.375 (we use 1.375 because she works out 3 days per week) = 2,019.2 calories per day with activity.

If she wants to lose a little weight and inches, we would subtract 250 calories to equal 1,769.2 calories per day. Then, if she burns another 250 calories per day through exercise, she will lose 1 to 2 pounds per week and have a total calorie intake of 1,519.2, which is still above her BMR of 1468.5. Make sense?

As this person reduces in size, she will redo her calculations. Once she hits her goal size, then she will calculate her BMR plus activity and eat that many calories each day to maintain. When you do the math, it becomes easy to maintain your ideal size once you reach your goal.

Now, let's calculate your BMR.

Women

655 + (4.35 × _____ lbs.) + (4.7 × _____ in.) – (4.7 × _____ age)

= _____ MY BMR

My BMR _____ × my activity level _____

= _____ My caloric intake to maintain, or AMR.

My caloric intake to maintain _____ – 250

= _____ My caloric intake for healthy weight and inches loss.

(I must still exercise to burn an additional 250 calories that day.)

Men

66 + (6.23 × _____ lbs.) + (12.7 × _____ in.) – (6.8 × _____ age)

= _____ MY BMR

My BMR _____ × my activity level _____

= _____ My caloric intake to maintain, or AMR.

My caloric intake to maintain _____ – 250

= _____ My caloric intake for healthy weight and inches loss.

(I must still exercise to burn an additional 250 calories that day.)

A FOOD LOG? I HAVE TO WRITE STUFF DOWN?

Now that we've looked up the calories in all of our favorite foods and beverages, let's start keeping track by physically writing down what you eat on paper, on your phone, or on your computer. Figure out which format will work best for you. I found that a little notepad in my purse worked well for me. I've had clients use spreadsheets or a fancy, spiral-bound diary. Others have used sticky notes—many, many sticky notes that were thrown around in a purse and then eventually stuck back together in some sort of order. (Oh, wait . . . I was the one who did that!) Where you choose to keep your food log doesn't matter as long as you put your newfound counting skills to use.

At first, you really do have to write down what you eat and drink. When you're a pro, you won't have to think about it because it will become second nature. Again, we are going for a *lifestyle* change here—without going bonkers!

There are two options you can choose from to keep a food log:

Option 1: The Not-Too-Much-Effort Option

This option involves keeping track of what you eat for one week. Only one week—that's it! Anybody can do anything for a week!

Option 2: The I'm-Really-Serious-about-Finally-Getting-to-the-Size-I-Want-to-Be-so-I'll-Choose-This-Option Option

Chances are, if you originally chose Option 1, you will find that what you wrote down was *so amazingly helpful* during that one little week that you want to keep the momentum. So, Option 2 is that you continue to write down what you consume each day until you finally reach your goals. That's it!

Some questions you may be asking at this point are:

- What sort of information should I keep in my food log?
- Do I have to get really technical and keep track of every little detail?

Again, I like to keep this as simple as possible. I think the most important items to keep track of are:

- Time of day
- Calories
- Fiber

- Protein
- Sodium
- Mood (optional)

If you want to keep it *super simple* at first, you can just keep track of three things: the *time of day* you eat (which will become very important in our next chapter, "Eat More ... and Eat More Frequently!"), type of food/beverage, and the *number of calories* consumed.

The super-simple food log option

- Time of day
- Type of food/beverage consumed
- Calories

If you want to add another level of challenge, you can start keeping track of the *fiber* and *protein* you eat as well.

Fiber

Fiber is important because it helps keep you feeling fuller longer, and it also keeps your system healthy. *Women should aim for 28 grams of fiber a day and men should aim for 35 grams a day.* You can find the fiber content on the nutrition label of any food item. Fiber helps lower LDL ("bad cholesterol"), helps keep blood sugar levels stable, helps keep you regular, and helps you lose inches. The calorie content of fiber actually doesn't count in your system because it's pushing everything through you. So ... fiber is your friend.

There are two types of fiber: *soluble* and *insoluble*.

Soluble fiber slows down digestion by attracting water in the system and forming a gel. This helps you feel fuller longer, which can help with losing inches. Some examples of soluble fiber are fruits like apples, pears, oranges, bananas, strawberries, blueberries, and raspberries. Other examples are vegetables like cucumbers, celery, beets, peas, and carrots. Lentils, oatmeal, barley, flaxseed, and beans are also examples of soluble fiber. There are many different types of beans such as black beans, black-eyed peas, kidney beans, garbanzo beans, pinto beans, lentils, lima beans, fava beans, and navy beans.

Insoluble fiber, including whole grains, whole wheat, barley, and brown rice, does not attract water in the body, so it goes right through you and keeps your gut healthy. Other examples of insoluble fiber are broccoli, zucchini, cauliflower, cabbage, onions, green beans, dark leafy greens, and the skins of root vegetables, like potato skins. Overall, you don't have to take a fiber supplement to get your fiber. Just eat your fruits, veggies, beans, and whole grains.

Protein

Protein is important because, well, we need protein, period! We need it for our organs, hair, skin, nails, muscles, our overall energy level, and for that toned look we desire. Protein helps you maintain any muscle that you currently have, and it helps build more muscle from exercise. Protein helps keep our blood sugar stable so we don't have energy highs and lows during the day. Adding protein to a meal also helps a person feel satiated. Examples of protein are eggs, chicken, fish, turkey, lean beef, and beans. ("Week 6: Fat, Protein, and Carbs" will go into more detail about protein.) I have found that if you are eating enough fiber and protein, you will naturally eat less of the other two values we haven't touched on yet, which are fat grams and carbohydrates (carbs). If you want to get really technical, you can keep track of everything, including fat and carbs.

Sodium

Sodium may also be something you want to keep track of, particularly if you are very water-retentive or have high blood pressure. Sodium is basically salt (or sodium chloride) added to food. We need a little bit of sodium in our diet to keep our body functioning properly. However, most people consume a ridiculous amount of sodium. The USDA currently recommends consumption of 2,300 mg of sodium per day or less. It also says that people with high blood pressure should aim for less than 1,500 mg per day. I personally know that if I ate that much sodium each day, I would be *very, very* bloated and water-retentive. I can always tell if I had too much salt in one day because I wake up the next morning and my upper eyelids are very, very puffy from water retention.

When I look at a food label, I aim for 300 mg or less of sodium per serving. If I put salt on my food when cooking, I only use a tiny bit of sea salt, which is also rich in minerals. I have noticed that when clients watch their sodium intake, they immediately lose several pounds of water weight. Why is that, you may ask? When a person has too much sodium, the body becomes dehydrated. So, it holds on to every drop of water that it can from beverages and food that you ingest. When you drink more water and reduce the sodium, the body doesn't have to hold on to as much water weight anymore because it is more hydrated. Our bodies are made of about 60 to 75 percent water. *All* of our cells need water to survive and function properly! So, reduce your sodium intake if you feel you are retaining too much water weight. Foods that are high in sodium include fast food, chips, french fries, hot dogs, soups, lunch meat, bacon, sausage, food in restaurants, cheese, and frozen meals. Start looking at the sodium content on food labels. You will be amazed at how much sodium is in certain foods.

I recently bought a quick sandwich at the airport when running to a flight. I didn't even look at the label because I was in a rush. When I was on the plane, I finally took out the sandwich and was excited to eat it because I was so hungry. *Then*, I looked at the label. It had 1,860 mg of sodium in it!! In one little sandwich! Needless to say, I only had a few bites, threw the rest away, and was very hungry (and very thirsty, thanks to the sodium I ingested) for the rest of the flight. I have since made it a practice to *always* look at the food labels in airports, even when I'm running late for a flight.

Mood

One final note—an interesting twist that you may want to consider tracking as part of your food log is your *mood* before and after every meal. Were you starving before you ate? Were you in a bad mood, so you ate too much at dinner? Did you have a stressful day, so you felt the need to consume two glasses of wine and a bar of chocolate right after work? All of these emotional notations will help you quite a bit in the long run, but again, keep things as simple as possible at the beginning. Your food log will soon be your BFF!

What format will your food log take? Online or paper? Here are a couple of handy pages to get you started during your first week (pages 26–29). You can also download them from my website: www.happyhealthypeople.com.

SUPER-SIMPLE FOOD LOG

Day	Time of Day		Type of Food/Beverage Consumed	Calories
Monday	Meal 1:	AM PM		
	Meal 2:	AM PM		
	Meal 3:	AM PM		
	Meal 4:	AM PM		
	Meal 5:	AM PM		
	Meal 6: (optional)	AM PM		
Tuesday	Meal 1:	AM PM		
	Meal 2:	AM PM		
	Meal 3:	AM PM		
	Meal 4:	AM PM		
	Meal 5:	AM PM		
	Meal 6: (optional)	AM PM		
Wednesday	Meal 1:	AM PM		
	Meal 2:	AM PM		
	Meal 3:	AM PM		
	Meal 4:	AM PM		
	Meal 5:	AM PM		
	Meal 6: (optional)	AM PM		
Thursday	Meal 1:	AM PM		
	Meal 2:	AM PM		
	Meal 3:	AM PM		

Day	Time of Day		Type of Food/Beverage Consumed	Calories
Thursday *(continued)*	Meal 4:	AM PM		
	Meal 5:	AM PM		
	Meal 6: *(optional)*	AM PM		
Friday	Meal 1:	AM PM		
	Meal 2:	AM PM		
	Meal 3:	AM PM		
	Meal 4:	AM PM		
	Meal 5:	AM PM		
	Meal 6: *(optional)*	AM PM		
Saturday	Meal 1:	AM PM		
	Meal 2:	AM PM		
	Meal 3	AM PM		
	Meal 4:	AM PM		
	Meal 5:	AM PM		
	Meal 6: *(optional)*	AM PM		
Sunday	Meal 1:	AM PM		
	Meal 2:	AM PM		
	Meal 3:	AM PM		
	Meal 4:	AM PM		
	Meal 5:	AM PM		
	Meal 6: *(optional)*	AM PM		

COMPLETE FOOD LOG
Here is an example of a more in-depth food log you can use.

Day	Time of Day		Type of Food/ Beverage Consumed	Calories	Fiber	Protein	Sodium	Mood
Monday	Meal 1:	AM PM						
	Meal 2:	AM PM						
	Meal 3:	AM PM						
	Meal 4:	AM PM						
	Meal 5:	AM PM						
	Meal 6: *(optional)*	AM PM						
Tuesday	Meal 1:	AM PM						
	Meal 2:	AM PM						
	Meal 3:	AM PM						
	Meal 4:	AM PM						
	Meal 5:	AM PM						
	Meal 6: *(optional)*	AM PM						
Wednesday	Meal 1:	AM PM						
	Meal 2:	AM PM						
	Meal 3:	AM PM						
	Meal 4:	AM PM						
	Meal 5:	AM PM						
	Meal 6: *(optional)*	AM PM						
Thursday	Meal 1:	AM PM						
	Meal 2:	AM PM						
	Meal 3:	AM PM						

Day	Time of Day		Type of Food/ Beverage Consumed	Calories	Fiber	Protein	Sodium	Mood
Thursday *(continued)*	Meal 4:	AM PM						
	Meal 5:	AM PM						
	Meal 6: *(optional)*	AM PM						
Friday	Meal 1:	AM PM						
	Meal 2:	AM PM						
	Meal 3:	AM PM						
	Meal 4:	AM PM						
	Meal 5:	AM PM						
	Meal 6: *(optional)*	AM PM						
Saturday	Meal 1:	AM PM						
	Meal 2:	AM PM						
	Meal 3	AM PM						
	Meal 4:	AM PM						
	Meal 5:	AM PM						
	Meal 6: *(optional)*	AM PM						
Sunday	Meal 1:	AM PM						
	Meal 2:	AM PM						
	Meal 3:	AM PM						
	Meal 4:	AM PM						
	Meal 5:	AM PM						
	Meal 6: *(optional)*	AM PM						

READING LABELS

Now that you know how many calories to aim for each day, I think it is important for me to teach you how to read a food label. Here is an example of the nutrition label for a grilled chicken Caesar salad at a chain restaurant. If you think a salad is healthy, think again!

Nutrition Facts
Serving Size 1 order 280g (280g)

Amount Per Serving

Calories 308   **Calories** from Fat 108

	% Daily Value*
Total Fat 12g	**21%**
Saturated Fat 4g	**17%**
Trans Fat	
Cholesterol 82mg	**39%**
Sodium 1298mg	**28%**
Total Carbohydrate 17g	**4%**
Dietary Fiber 3g	**4%**
Sugars 4g	
Protein 33g	

Vitamin A 111% • **Vitamin C** 40%

Calcium 41% • **Iron** 9%

*Percent Daily Values are based on a 2,000 calorie diet. Your daily values may be higher or lower depending on your calorie needs:

		Calories	2,000	2,500
Total Fat	Less Than		65g	80g
Saturated Fat	Less Than		20g	25g
Cholesterol	Less Than		300mg	300mg
Sodium	Less Than		2,400mg	2,400mg
Total Carbohydrate			300g	375g
Dietary Fiber			25g	30g

Calories per gram:
Fat 9 • Carbohydrate 4 • Protein 4

When you first look at a nutrition label, it is important to start at the top. In this case, the "serving size" is one order, because it is a salad. When you look at the label on a bag of chips, for example, pay attention to the serving size! It may say that ten chips are 150 calories, but there are *three servings per bag*. So then you would have to *triple* each number on the food label. Instead of eating 150 calories, you are actually eating 450!

There are a total of 308 calories in this salad. Seems healthy, right? Let's keep reading. There is no trans fat, which is good. The cholesterol is low, which is also good. However, let's look at the sodium. There are 1,298 mg of sodium in this salad. Wow! That's a lot of sodium! As I said, I try to keep sodium to 300 mg or *less* per serving when I look at food labels. Too much sodium causes water retention and high blood pressure.

The carbs in this salad are relatively low, at 17 grams. There are 3 grams of fiber and there is very little sugar, at 4 grams. It is also very high in protein, at 33 grams. So, there are good points and bad points to this salad. Probably the chicken and salad dressing are what cause the sodium to be so high. So, it is better to make your own grilled chicken Caesar salad at home, because then you can control what you put in it.

One simple way to stay within your calorie range is to eat appropriate portion sizes. Here is an easy way to remember how to measure portions:

- 3 oz. meat/fish/poultry = a deck of cards or the palm of your hand
- 1 cup = a baseball or the size of your fist
- ½ cup = computer mouse
- 1 teaspoon = tip of the thumb
- 1 oz. = 2 dice
- 2 tablespoons = a golf ball

BABY GOALS AND BABY STEPS

Now that you've figured out exactly how much you should be consuming to lose inches the healthy way and you know how to read a food label, it is time to set our baby goals for the week. You can use some of the same goals from last week if you feel you haven't mastered them yet. Or, we can create brand new goals right here.

Some sample baby goals for this week are:

1. I will look up the calories of my favorite foods and beverages.
2. I will start writing down what I eat and the time of day on a little notepad or on my phone.
3. I will calculate my caloric intake for inches loss and keep a food log.

You get the picture. Just write down three goals that you know you can stick to for this week. Go by what "feels easy" for you to do; then you'll be sure to keep them!

My three baby goals for this week are:

1. _____

_____

2. _____

_____

3. _____

_____

Before we conclude this chapter, let's take another round of measurements, shall we? I know, I know: You've just begun counting your calories and recording them in a food log. You just figured out your ideal daily caloric intake. Still, it is important to continue this measurement habit. Besides, my guess is that you will already start to see a difference in just one week by being more aware of your daily food habits.

Celebrate losing even as little as a quarter inch in any area! Rather than a celebratory meal, treat yourself to a spa treatment or a shopping trip. You should be proud of yourself for taking control of your life and your health and doing it in a way that will create sustainable lifestyle changes. We want to take baby steps to lose your inches. That way they will stay off!

Week 2 Measurements

_____ Waist (1 in. above belly button)

_____ Hips (widest part around glutes)

_____ Lower abdomen (2 in. below BB)

_____ Right thigh (put right hand flat against leg and measure under the thumb area)

_____ Left thigh (put left hand flat against leg and measure under the thumb area)

_____ Chest (measure around widest part)

_____ Right arm (measure around bicep area)

_____ Left arm (measure around bicep area)

_____ Right calf (measure around widest part)

_____ Left calf (measure around widest part)

_____ INCHES LOST THIS WEEK

_____ CHANGE SINCE LAST WEEK

_____ TOTAL INCHES LOST SO FAR

WEEK 3

Eat More ... and Eat More Frequently!

How to *Not* Lose Your Mind: Lesson for Week 3

You should never starve yourself to try to lose inches and pounds! In fact, eating too little leads to health problems and eventually **crazy weight gain**. Plus, if you starve yourself, then all you can think about is food and it can make you feel nutty!

This chapter is to teach you that there is a right way and a wrong way to lose weight and inches. I'm here to show you the right way so that your waistline shrinks and you maintain your sanity.

THE ACCIDENTAL ANOREXIC

Earlier I warned you that there would be stories about me in this book. Here is a story from a time when I knew nothing about anything regarding weight loss and dieting. When I first started out on my journey to lose the weight I put on in college, I saw a women's magazine in the grocery store that said "Lose weight by eating only 1,200 calories a day!" Good idea, right? *Wrong.* I then bought one of the little books, also at the grocery checkout counter, that listed the calorie content of every type of food. (Note—this was *before* anything technologically fancy or the word "online" even existed.) By counting my calories and exercising, I was beginning to move toward my goal of a leaner, trimmer body.

The first 10 pounds fell off easily. I looked better, I felt better, and I began to wonder: What would happen if I ate *less than* 1,200 calories a day? Wouldn't I lose weight faster? That's how I became an "accidental anorexic" for two months. The key word here is "accidental" because

I really had no idea what I was doing. Anorexia is not something that should be taken lightly, so it's my job to make sure you lose your inches the healthy way.

I didn't think of myself as an anorexic at that time. I had no idea that your body needs a minimum number of calories to survive for basic bodily functions, like breathing and keeping your heart beating. I thought further restricting my consumption of food would simply help me lose weight faster. I didn't know my body would rebel.

So now my innocent journey takes a not-so-good twist. I began to keep a food log—just as I am recommending you do—but as I recorded every bite, I got increasingly overzealous. I took note of how many calories were in each forkful. My daily caloric intake kept getting smaller: From 1,200 calories, I went to 800 calories, then 500, 400, and 300. I know, I know . . . it seriously makes me cringe to think about it now. But back then, I had no idea what I was doing to myself.

You might ask, "How could a smart girl be so silly?" Shouldn't I have known it was too little food to keep myself alive and healthy? You would think so, but I really had no clue. I lost weight, but it was not the right type of weight loss—it was muscle weight (think: no toning and no strength at all). By the end of the summer, I was skeletally skinny. At the same time, my menstrual cycle stopped, my skin looked dull, my nails were breaking, and my hair started falling out—the exact opposite of the attractive look I was hoping to achieve. By the way, ladies, unless you are in menopause, any time your menstrual cycle stops, it is really bad. That is your body's way of trying to preserve your life by slowly shutting down basic bodily functions because you are starving yourself.

Now some of you reading this right now are thinking, "I am totally going to do what she did. I don't care if she says not to. She got skinny, so what's the big deal?" Not so fast! What followed my getting "skinny" was a period of crisis in which I drew the attention (fortunately) of my parents, and a recovery that included gaining back every single pound *plus more*. I actually ended up *heavier* than I started, because when your body is starving, it will hold on to every morsel of food for dear life once you start eating like a normal human being. In fact, what happened is that I gained 45 pounds and four sizes in four months. That is how fast the weight packed back on when I resumed eating normal portions. So, I became heavier than I was before I started, and I had to go back to square one. This time, I'll do it the healthy way.

EAT MORE!

Experiences like the one I just described led me on the path to figure out how to lose inches the healthy way and keep them off. As hard as some of my past experiences were, I am grateful, because they guided me to become a health coach and nutritionist and enabled me to help others.

One of the most fascinating things that I have learned in my practice is that most of my clients do not eat enough nor frequently enough. The most ironic thing is that usually the people who need to lose the *most* actually eat the *least*. I know that some of you are saying "Yeah, right," as you read this, but it's the truth. The people who need to lose the most decide to go on a "diet." This diet typically involves not eating breakfast or just highly caffeinating themselves when they wake up, running out the door, not eating anything until noon, having a microscopic lunch (if any lunch at all), and then having a "healthy" dinner. This may make them reach a grand total of one half of the calories they actually need to be eating during the day. As a result of this not-eating-enough plan, these individuals can't lose a single pound. In fact, they may even *gain* a few pounds, because their bodies are rebelling!

Ladies and gentlemen, from my experience with coaching others, I can say that no matter what size you are at this moment, if your daily meal plan even slightly resembles what I just described, you actually need to *eat more* if you want your pants to start falling off of you. Let me tell you why...

During the hunter-gatherer period of time, if our ancestors didn't hunt and kill their food that day, they didn't eat. Plain and simple. The body is really an amazing creation; it is designed to survive in almost any situation, including prolonged periods of little or no food. This means that when your body is in starvation mode, it thinks that there is a famine going on in the world and it may never see food again. When the body is not getting enough food to operate at peak capacity, it slows the metabolism way down. It does that to preserve the fat, or "fuel," that we have stored in our bodies. When we DO find food during this "famine period," the body will store the food you eat as *fat*, just in case it never sees another meal again. So, our metabolism is slowing down, our bodies are storing nourishment as fat to survive, and in our brains, we somehow think it makes sense to starve ourselves to lose weight. Really?

If our body could sit down and have a conversation with our brain and discuss all the little tricks and mind games we play on ourselves, our bodies would be so very, very confused. Our bodies would probably say "Do you mean to tell me there is more food out there than you are giving me? Why in the world are you torturing me? *Feed me, please*, and I'll release some of this fat I've been storing around your middle and in your love handles!"

A simpler conversation may go like this:

Brain to Body: "I've decided to not eat enough so I can get skinny."

Body to Brain: "You're an idiot!"

Either way, I think you get my drift. The body only wants to survive. If you give it food, it will release its stored fat.

If you go longer than three hours without eating during the day, the body starts to go into "fasting mode" or "starvation mode." So, to prevent this from occurring, try to eat something every three hours. When you start this new habit, it takes a couple of weeks for your body to recognize that it will regularly be getting food and then speed up your metabolism. Soon you will notice you are hungrier more frequently, which means your metabolism has sped up.

I had a client lose 42 pounds in two months and 53 pounds in three months—simply by eating every three hours. She set a timer on her cell phone, and magic happened. She was in her fifties, a nurse, on her feet all day, and had to take care of her elderly parents when she got home. She didn't eat breakfast, she barely nibbled during the day because she wanted to lose weight, and she was too busy to eat. She claimed she was never hungry. Well, of course she wasn't, because her body was starving! Her metabolism had slowed down, which is why she wasn't very hungry, and every little thing she ate got stored as fat for survival. Needless to say, after a few weeks of working with me, she ate something every three hours and the fat just melted off. It was miraculous. She told me in a testimonial, "I wanted to thank you for the healthier me. Who knew I was accidentally starving myself! Now that I am following your advice daily, losing weight seems so easy!" I recently heard from her, and she has kept off a total of 62 pounds for over two years!

Her story is the perfect example of the body's natural starvation response and what can happen when you give it food every three hours. So, listen to your health coach: To "lose your inches without losing your mind," *eat more*, and those inches will melt away. When does eating more begin? It begins with breakfast.

BUT I'M NOT HUNGRY AT BREAKFAST!

I hear this excuse all the time. My response? *I don't care! Eat breakfast anyway!* We have all heard that breakfast is the most important meal of the day, and it is absolutely true. Breakfast wakes up your body and metabolism and gives you energy to start your day. Your metabolism is what burns calories all day long. You should aim to eat within 45 minutes of waking up. If you are currently skipping breakfast, I don't care what you eat—just eat something within 45 minutes of waking: a boiled egg, some yogurt, a little organic peanut butter on toast, a banana, high-fiber cereal, some fruit...something—anything! See pages 40-41 for some quick and healthy breakfast ideas. There are also more breakfast ideas on my Mix-and-Match Meal Plan in Appendix II on page 169.

Think of your metabolism as a fireplace. When you are sleeping, it runs on embers—it is still burning, just at a much slower rate. When you eat breakfast, it puts logs on the fire. So, if you want to burn more calories throughout the day (and get slimmer), *eat something!* One day you will wake up actually feeling hungry for breakfast, and on this magical day, you will know that your metabolism has sped up.

For those of you who want to eat something relatively healthy for breakfast, focus on protein, complex carbs, and fiber. Eggs are great and easy to cook. I'll often eat a slice of high-fiber toast with one or two organic eggs. I use free-range organic eggs, mind you—more omega-3s and vitamin D. Plus, the chickens actually get to go outside and see the sunlight. I love oatmeal as well. I'll make one serving of plain oatmeal and swirl in 1 tablespoon of organic peanut butter and raw honey. Sometimes I'll add a little cinnamon. Delicious! The peanut butter gets all melted and gooey—I love it. This way, I'm getting complex carbs, fiber, protein, and healthy fats all at breakfast.

Want cold cereal? Great! Get a high-fiber cereal—some have as much as 14 grams of fiber per serving! Basically, the more fiber, the better. Use organic milk or, my favorites, unsweetened almond, cashew, or coconut milk. Yum! You can even vary between unsweetened chocolate and unsweetened vanilla almond milk. Maybe add some blueberries or strawberries to your cold cereal.

In a rush? Make a smoothie. Add some frozen berries and a scoop of plain Greek yogurt, or you can make a protein shake (I like to make a chocolate and peanut butter protein shake). In an even greater rush? Grab a protein bar. Get one that does not have artificial sweeteners or soy protein isolate in it and that has at least 10 grams of protein; 15 to 20 grams are even better.

Breakfast Ideas
- Plain oatmeal—add cinnamon, sliced banana, or raw honey if you'd like
- High-fiber cereal with unsweetened almond, cashew, coconut, or organic milk
- A slice of high-fiber toast with organic peanut or almond butter
- Greek yogurt—try adding fresh fruit and chia seeds
- Two free-range eggs with a slice of high-fiber toast and a little avocado or coconut oil spread

- Homemade breakfast sandwich—two slices of high-fiber bread, an egg, and low-sodium nitrate-free turkey bacon
- Cottage cheese with fruit
- Two hard-boiled eggs
- Fruit smoothie—plain Greek yogurt, a banana, and some frozen berries
- Chocolate, banana, and peanut butter protein shake (yum!). Take one to two scoops chocolate whey protein powder, ½ banana, one scoop organic peanut butter, ½–1 cup water or unsweetened almond milk and lots of ice. Blend and enjoy!
- Egg white omelet with veggies
- Scrambled eggs with a side of sliced avocado
- Protein bar—select one with no artificial sweeteners, no soy protein isolate, and 10 to 20 grams of protein (the more the better).

As you can see, there are many options for breakfast. I don't care which breakfast idea you choose to eat—just eat *something* within 45 minutes of waking.

So, what are you going to eat tomorrow morning? Look up the calories of your current favorites and make a list of five breakfasts you can eat that will give you an energetic boost without overloading you with calories.

There are several conflicting recommendations out there about how to portion your calories throughout the day. I think a good general recommendation is to have 20–25 percent of your calories at breakfast, the same at lunch, and the same at dinner. The two snacks in between should each be about 10–15 percent of your daily calories. So, if my daily calorie requirement is 1,500, then my breakfast, lunch, and dinner would be about 300–375 calories each, and my two snacks would be about 150–225 calories each. This way, your blood sugar will be balanced all day, and you should never feel like you are starving. You should have plenty of energy and never feel too full. Everyone's appetites are different, so you may find that a bigger breakfast, a medium-sized lunch, and a smaller dinner work best for you. In general, it's a good idea to eat dinner a few hours before bedtime so that the body has time to properly digest it before you go to sleep. Aim to eat dinner by 7:00 p.m., if you can.

My Top 5 Favorite Breakfast Foods

Food	Calories	Portion Size
1.		
2.		
3.		
4.		
5.		

WHY AM I STARVING BY DINNER?

This answer ties in to what we just learned—it's because you didn't have any breakfast! What I have noticed when I coach clients is that when they don't eat breakfast and they try to eat "good" all day—i.e., they don't eat enough—they are starving by dinner. Maybe you had a low-calorie cereal with skim milk for breakfast, you ate a piece of fruit as a snack, you skipped lunch, and now it's dinnertime and you are starving. You know what? This is literally true, because you did not eat enough calories during the day to sustain a small puppy.

When you don't eat enough all day, you may find that as you start to prepare dinner for either yourself or your family, your hand magically keeps putting food into your mouth while getting the meal ready. "It's okay, I was 'good' all day," you say to yourself. Soon enough, dinner is ready and you're not feeling too hungry, but the family is waiting, so you eat more with them. After dinner, you are craving something sweet (perfectly normal, by the way. I always have a few chocolate chips after dinner; see page 174 for some healthy dessert ideas). You have that secret pint of no-fat-not-too-much-taste-low-calorie ice cream in the freezer, so you help yourself to a few scoops after dinner. A few scoops turns into a half pint, and half of a pint turns into just a few frozen crumbs left at the bottom of the container. But, you were "good" all day, so it's okay, right?

The problem with being "good" all day is that you are really just playing mind games with your brain—and your body isn't buying it. When you deprive yourself all day and only allow yourself these tiny little morsels of food, your body rebels: "Brain, you are *crazy*! I'm going to eat now because I'm starving, and there's nothing you can do about it!" This, incidentally, is when you'll have your late-night cravings, usually for sweets and simple carbs.

Eat More Frequently

The trick to not eating too much before, during, and after dinner is to *eat more food during the day*. That's right! It's okay to add an egg or two with breakfast, or have *two* pieces of fruit as a snack, or even add some almonds during the day. If you eat larger portions during the day, you will feel more satisfied at night and won't feel the need to bond with a pint of ice cream. Try it. Your body and especially your brain will thank you. To end those mind games, eat more during the day.

Not only do we need to eat more food, but we also need to *eat more frequently* throughout the day. I mentioned earlier that most of the people I coach do not eat frequently enough. Changing this habit alone can easily get you to the size you want to be.

I think we've all heard that we should eat small meals, five to six times a day. We've read it in magazines and heard it on the news. So why didn't we do it? Maybe we didn't understand the concept. Now that we know we need to eat regularly to keep our metabolism performing at optimal speed, we should finally be convinced this is an ideal way to eat. You want to eat every two to three hours. After that three-hour mark, your body starts to go into that "starvation mode" we discussed previously.

Some clients tell me they forget to eat, and that is why they go longer than three hours without eating. My solution? Set an alarm. Use your cell phone or a kitchen timer, or set the alarm on your watch. Remind yourself to eat—your body will thank you later.

Let's take a minute to determine the times during the day you are probably waiting too long to eat. When do you need to fit in that extra snack? Below I have noted five "meals," so a meal/snack every three hours over fifteen hours gets us to the five meals a day. I also included the time you wake up, so you can see how long after waking you are waiting to eat breakfast. Fill in the approximate time you eat each meal in the following chart:

When Do I Eat Currently?	Time
I wake up at:	
Meal 1 Breakfast:	
Meal 2 Snack:	
Meal 3 Lunch:	
Meal 4 Snack:	
Meal 5 Dinner:	

If you are currently not eating five meals a day, that's okay. Just fill in the times of the meals you are currently eating

Now, what changes do you need to make to your eating schedule? Write your *new* eating schedule in this chart so that you can burn those calories at peak capacity all day long!

My New Eating Schedule	Time
I wake up at:	
Meal 1 Breakfast:	
Meal 2 Snack:	
Meal 3 Lunch:	
Meal 4 Snack:	
Meal 5 Dinner:	

A sample before-and-after eating schedule may look like this:

Before	Time	After	Time
I wake up at:	6:00 a.m.	I wake up at:	6:00 a.m.
Meal 1 Breakfast:	none	Meal 1 Breakfast:	6:30 a.m.
Meal 2 Snack:	9:00 a.m.	Meal 2 Snack:	9:00 a.m.
Meal 3 Lunch:	12:00 p.m.	Meal 3 Lunch:	12:00 p.m.
Meal 4 Snack:	none	Meal 4 Snack:	3:00 p.m.
Meal 5 Dinner:	6:00 p.m.	Meal 5 Dinner:	6:00 p.m.

BABY GOALS AND BABY STEPS

Let's wrap up Week 3 with our by-now-familiar baby goals and inches measurement. Isn't it wonderful how these baby goals are starting to become second nature? Keep going! You're doing great!

Some sample baby goals for this week are:

1. I will eat breakfast within 45 minutes of waking.
2. I will eat every three hours.
3. I will bring healthy snacks to work and store them in the office refrigerator.

My three baby goals for this week are:

1. _____

   _____

2. _____

   _____

3. _____

   _____

It's time to take your measurements! Let's see how you did this week:

Week 3 Measurements

_____ Waist (1 in. above belly button)

_____ Hips (widest part around glutes)

_____ Lower abdomen (2 in. below BB)

_____ Right thigh (put right hand flat against leg and measure under the thumb area)

_____ Left thigh (put left hand flat against leg and measure under the thumb area)

_____ Chest (measure around widest part)

_____ Right arm (measure around bicep area)

_____ Left arm (measure around bicep area)

_____ Right calf (measure around widest part)

_____ Left calf (measure around widest part)

_____ INCHES LOST THIS WEEK

_____ CHANGE SINCE LAST WEEK

_____ TOTAL INCHES LOST SO FAR

WEEK 4
Now MOVE IT!

MYTHS OF METABOLISM

It is not necessarily true that your metabolism slows down as you get older. Thermogenesis, or the part of the metabolism that processes food, actually stays about the same as we age. What is true is that as we get older, we tend to become more sedentary. Many people have desk jobs, we tend to become less active as we age, and sometimes it seems easier to relax on the couch rather than to go exercise. As individuals become more sedentary, they lose muscle mass, store more fat, and their BMR (basal metabolic rate) decreases, so they burn fewer calories. That is why people think metabolism slows down as we age. It is okay to relax and watch TV, but it is important to stay active as well. Now that I'm a little older, being active is essential to keep my inches off. I remember I had one very inspirational member of my gym—a woman who was ninety-six years old. She worked out three times a week, still could drive herself, was in great shape, and had tons of energy. To me, she was the perfect example of how we don't necessarily have to let our metabolism slow down as we age.

I first discovered the importance of exercise (and what happens when it is lacking) my freshman year at Notre Dame. In high school, for example, I never packed on the pounds, despite eating whatever I wanted, simply because I was so active. During the fall, I marched it off during band practice, and in the spring, I played softball. When I got to Notre Dame, I was still playing the clarinet in the marching band, so I got a decent amount of exercise in the fall semester (yes, I will forever be a band dork, by the way).

When I returned to school after the winter break my freshman year, I had eaten too many Christmas goodies with no real exercise, and I had put on a good 5 to 10 pounds. Most of my clothes still fit, so that was okay, right? Everyone has heard of the "freshman fifteen," after all. I often visited the campus hangout, which was aptly named "La Fun." This student hangout literally had a Wall of Candy as well as pizza, chips, and fast food. The school dining hall had twenty kinds of sugar cereals, french fries, mozzarella sticks, fried chicken tenders, frozen yogurt (called "yo-cream"), cookies . . . you can see where this is going.

I was very inactive in the spring semester, and by the time my freshman year was over, I had gained 25 pounds of pure blubber. It wasn't that my metabolism had changed all of a sudden; only one year had passed, and I was still nineteen years old! Rather, it was all of that late-night eating, dining hall food, and not being very active that had caught up with me. I couldn't kid myself anymore or make up any more excuses—everything in my closet was tight—I was 25 pounds heavier than when I started college. There was nothing left to do when I returned home but to drop the weight. And to do that, I had to get back into exercise.

Simple Q & A

Do you have to move your body to "lose your inches"? **YES.**

Will you lose some inches just by watching what you eat? **YES.**

Will you be able to lose all the inches that you want just by watching what you eat? **NO.**

Can you get that toned look that every woman and man strives for just by watching what you eat? **NO.**

Do you have to move your body in order to re-shape and re-tone your body? **YES!**

GET READY TO MOVE IT

Now, I know some of you are having an anxiety attack at the thought of entering a gym, let alone joining one! Fear not, dear ones. There are a number of ways to get the exercise you need to lose those inches.

When I first started exercising, I would walk 45 minutes every day around my neighborhood while holding these little 1-pound hand weights that my mom had. I then used exercise DVDs in the comfort of my home. Since then, I've taken boot camp classes, kickboxing, body sculpting, boxing, spinning, CrossFit, and all kinds of other classes. Today, I am a Certified Personal Trainer. Before I was certified, I worked with several personal trainers throughout the years and was a member of several gyms. So, you see, there are *many* options for you to ease into exercising. We will work together to figure out which one will work best for you.

Before engaging in any exercise program, it is important to check with your doctor to make sure you follow an exercise program that is right for you. The US Department of Agriculture (USDA) has come up with several guidelines regarding exercise for weight loss and weight maintenance. The USDA says

- Adults between the ages of eighteen and sixty-four should have at least 2½ hours each week of aerobic physical activity at a moderate level OR 1 hour and 15 minutes of aerobic physical activity at a vigorous level.
- Being active five or more hours each week can provide even more health benefits.

- You should spread aerobic activity out over at least three days a week.
- Each activity should be done for at least 10 minutes at a time.
- Adults should also do strengthening activities, like push-ups, sit-ups, and lifting weights, at least two days a week.

Now, upon reading that for the first time, it just seems confusing. In a nutshell, you should do 30 minutes of aerobic physical activity (cardio) at least three times a week and resistance training at least two times a week. Resistance training is also referred to as strength training or lifting weights. Here are some examples of cardio and resistance training:

Examples of Cardio

- Walking
- Running
- Jogging
- Swimming
- Elliptical
- Stair climbing
- Cycling
- Jumping rope
- Boxing
- Spinning
- Kickboxing
- Zumba®

Examples of Resistance Training

- Weight machines
- Taking a sculpting or toning class in a gym
- Exercise DVDs that use weights and full-body exercises
- Circuit training
- Dumbbells
- Barbells
- CrossFit
- Push-ups, lunges, squats, and other full-body exercises that only use body weight

Exercising five days a week may be the easiest way for you to keep track. A sample exercise schedule for five days a week would look like this:

Monday: Cardio (30 minutes)

Tuesday: Resistance training (30 minutes)

Wednesday: Cardio (30 minutes)

Thursday: Resistance training (30 minutes)

Friday: Cardio (30 minutes)

Saturday: Rest or light walk

Sunday: Rest

You may not have time to exercise five days a week, so let's compile everything into three days a week to start. Again, baby steps! A three-day-a-week exercise schedule may look like this:

Monday: Full-body circuit workout plus cardio (30–60 minutes)

Tuesday: Rest

Wednesday: Full-body circuit workout plus cardio (30–60 minutes)

Thursday: Rest

Friday: Full-body circuit workout plus cardio (30–60 minutes)

Saturday: Rest

Sunday: Rest

Or, if it has been years since you've worked out or you are just getting back into exercise, a simpler beginning workout schedule might look like this:

Monday: Walk (30–60 minutes)

Tuesday: Rest

Wednesday: Walk (30–60 minutes)

Thursday: Rest

Friday: Walk (30–60 minutes)

Saturday: Rest

Sunday: Rest

If exercising is extremely new to you or if you haven't exercised in a while, you can even break up the 30 minutes into two 15-minute increments. So, you can exercise 15 minutes in the morning and 15 minutes at lunch or in the evening to get in your 30 minutes a day. Feel free to start with walking as your form of exercise and build up to a more challenging routine.

When I owned a gym, we would often do a promotion where a person had to do a 30-minute workout three days a week for twenty-one days. We measured them before and after the twenty-one days. The reason for the twenty-one days is a principle discovered by Dr. Maxwell Maltz in 1960 that it takes twenty-one days to make a habit. We had hundreds and hundreds of individuals do this promotion. Guess what happened? *One hundred percent of them lost inches.* Every single time, without fail. I'm not kidding!! That's how I got the idea for this book!

Our 30-minute workout consisted of cardio and resistance training at the same time, which was very efficient and produced obvious results. After the promotion, however, some of our members decided to change it up—or they just got too busy (or too lazy!)—and decided to work out only two days a week. A few months later they would come to me and say, "Justine, why am I not losing anymore?" And I would say, "Well, how often are you coming in here each week?" Then they would say, "Well, twice a week because . . . " at which point I would cut them off and say, "There's the issue. You have to do three times a week! Three times a week is the magic number. So, figure out what you can do in your schedule to get here that third day."

Do you want to know something fascinating? When they incorporated that third day back into their weekly workout routine, they *lost inches again*! Without fail, every single time. This whole process was like a big science experiment to me—it was fascinating! So, now I always tell everyone, "Three times a week is the magic number!"

Obviously, if you can work out more often, great, but to start, I think three times a week is the perfect number and can easily fit into your schedule.

YOUR EXERCISE SCHEDULE

Let's look at your schedule and see where you can squeeze in your 30 minutes. Now, we may have to set aside an hour, just in case you are commuting to a gym or a class. But, if you are working out at home, outside, or with a buddy, then you can probably set aside closer to half an hour. Write down your current exercise schedule in the following chart.

For example, 15-minute walk on Monday, Wednesday, and Friday at lunch around the office building. Or, 20 minutes on the elliptical every single morning after I wake up. It's also okay if you put "none."

MY CURRENT EXERCISE SCHEDULE

Day	Activity	Time (Duration)
Monday		
Tuesday		
Wednesday		
Thursday		
Friday		
Saturday		
Sunday		

Now, look at what you are doing. Is it just cardio? Is it just resistance training? Are you able to do anything consistently? Do you even *like* the form of exercise you are currently doing, or do you want to try something new? I think it's really important that you enjoy what you're

doing, both in terms of being able to stick to it and being able to progress slowly within the exercise program that is right for you. Now let's
total how many hours and minutes you are active each week:

- I currently am getting _____ hours and _____ minutes of
  cardio a week.
- I currently am getting _____ hours and _____ minutes of
  resistance training a week.
- I like / don't like what I'm doing. (circle one)
- I want to fit in more cardio / resistance training / both
  into my schedule. (circle one)

We need to make sure you are getting cardio *and* resistance training. Most people are able to do cardio, which will increase your heart
health and increase your overall energy level, in addition to reducing
your inches. Resistance training can be a tougher sell, most notably for
two reasons. The first is the objection, which we encountered in Week
1, that doing resistance or strength training ("weights") will actually
bulk you up and produce the opposite result from losing inches.

As we discussed earlier, this is simply not true. To avoid becoming
a "skinny-fat person," which we now know is not an ideal look, a person has to do resistance training and lift weights. This doesn't mean
huffing and puffing and grunting in the gym—which by the way is the
second objection that most people have to resistance training—they
think it means hanging out by the big, sweaty, muscle guys with no
neck. Instead, it means doing squats, lunges, push-ups (on the knees
or regular), and bicep curls. It could also mean using an exercise DVD
that incorporates weights or bands, OR it means attending a fitness
class that does something with weights *and* cardio, OR it means using
dumbbells when you work out at home, OR it means doing a nice circuit workout that a trainer shows you in your gym, OR it means just
getting your own personal trainer. As you can see, there are many ways
to incorporate resistance training into your life that are fun and easy
to follow.

Since we've been able to break down the exercise you're doing now, have found out a little bit more about what you like to do, and now know how much more you need, we can create a new exercise schedule for you. Be sure to give yourself at least one day of rest.

MY NEW EXERCISE SCHEDULE

Day	Activity	Time (Duration)
Monday		
Tuesday		
Wednesday		
Thursday		
Friday		
Saturday		
Sunday		

BABY GOALS AND BABY STEPS

Now that we've come up with your ideal exercise plan, I'm sure there are a couple of things you need to do to make those goals a reality. Do you need to join a gym? Do you need to call around to places that offer fitness classes and find out about pricing? Do you need to call a buddy to start planning your walks? Do you need to just walk out the front door and start taking your own walks?

Some sample baby goals for this week are:

1. I will start walking for 30 minutes a day on Monday, Wednesday, and Friday.
2. I will call local gyms to see what their prices are.
3. I will invite my friend to go visit the local gyms with me.

Take a moment to figure out the steps you need to take (again, baby steps!) to make your new, fabulous exercise schedule a reality!

My three baby goals for this week to create my new exercise schedule are:

1. _____

   _____

2. _____

   _____

3. _____

   _____

Wonderful! Now you have all of your baby goals in place. Let's wrap up Week 4 with our by-now-familiar inches measurement. You have done *amazing* so far and you should be very proud of yourself! Not too many people would stick to anything for one week, let alone four. You're also past the twenty-one-day mark, which means you are inadvertently creating healthy, sustainable habits! Keep it up! I'm proud of you!

Week 4 Measurements

_____ Waist (1 in. above belly button)

_____ Hips (widest part around glutes)

_____ Lower abdomen (2 in. below BB)

_____ Right thigh (put right hand flat against leg and measure under the thumb area)

_____ Left thigh (put left hand flat against leg and measure under the thumb area)

_____ Chest (measure around widest part)

_____ Right arm (measure around bicep area)

_____ Left arm (measure around bicep area)

_____ Right calf (measure around widest part)

_____ Left calf (measure around widest part)

_____ INCHES LOST THIS WEEK

_____ CHANGE SINCE LAST WEEK

_____ TOTAL INCHES LOST SO FAR

WEEK 5

Don't Drink Calories

Here's the deal: our bodies are made of mostly water—anywhere from 60 to 75 percent water depending on the day and body type, with adult males averaging slightly higher. Our brain tissue is made of approximately 85 percent water.[3] This means that each cell craves water every single day. The problem comes when many of us don't consume enough H_2O on a daily basis to keep our bodies at the peak of their game. Many of my clients don't realize they are very dehydrated on a day-to-day basis. When you are dehydrated, you actually retain water, which equals extra pounds and inches.

WE ARE WATER

How much water should you actually consume to keep your cells and your metabolism functioning properly? We've all heard the recommendation to drink eight glasses of water a day, or 64 ounces. This is a good general rule of thumb. The average water bottle size is 16 ounces, so that means you need to refill your water bottle four times a day to get your 64 ounces.

If you want to be more specific as far as calculating your water intake, the recommended Dietary Reference Intake (DRI) is 91 ounces total

---

3 Fereydoon Batmanghelidj, *Your Body's Many Cries for Water* (Falls Church, VA: Global Health Solutions, 2008), 6.

for a sedentary woman and 125 ounces total for a sedentary man. About 19 percent of total water intake comes from food, so subtracting that, a sedentary woman should have 74 ounces of water a day (9 cups) and a sedentary man should have 101 ounces per day (12 cups).

More active people, of course, need more water. The American Council of Sports Medicine recommends 13.5 to 20 ounces of water two to three hours before exercise and 5 to 12 ounces of water in 15- to 20-minute intervals during exercise. This means you should be drinking at least half of your water bottle, or better yet, *all* of your water bottle if you are doing a 60-minute workout session.

The key to all of this is to drink water *before* you get thirsty because, by the time you are thirsty, you are actually dehydrated! A good rule of thumb to check if you are dehydrated is to look at the color of your urine. Yes, I know what you're thinking, but it's true. The yellower it is, the more dehydrated you are. Your goal is for it to be clear and colorless—that's when you know you've had enough water.

OBJECTIONS TO DRINKING ENOUGH WATER

Now that you know why it's important to drink eight glasses of water a day, you need to examine your current daily water intake. Your body might be suffering a drought at this very minute! If you're like the rest of us, you may have some objections to drinking enough water. Let's go through some of the most common excuses for not drinking good ol' H_2O.

"I hate the taste. It's so boring!"
Give your water some all-natural flavor with a touch of lemon juice, a lime wedge, or an orange wedge. You can even add a slice of cucumber, cantaloupe, or honeydew to give it a refreshing taste.

"I forget to drink water during the day."

The easiest way to break this habit is to always carry a bottle of water with you. Have one in your car, on your desk, in your purse, or in your duffel bag. If a water bottle is in your sight, you will remember to drink from it. I never leave the house without one. The best thing is to get a refillable water bottle that is BPA free (BPA is bisphenol A, a chemical that may be toxic and is found in plastics). That way, you don't get the toxins while getting your H_2O.

"Won't I have to go to the restroom all the time?"

I recommend sipping water throughout the day, which allows you to get used to your increased water consumption without going to the restroom so often. If you drink one large glass of water in a matter of minutes to catch up on your water intake in one sitting, then you will have to go to the restroom shortly after. But if you drink smaller increments of water throughout the day instead, then your bladder won't get so overwhelmed.

"But I like those zero-calorie diet drinks. Don't they count?"

The nutrition labels on zero-calorie diet drinks can be pretty persuasive. When you take a closer look at what those chemistry lab-created artificial sweeteners are really doing to your body, however, you might not be quite so eager to pop the tab and start sipping faux sugar.

"What about seltzer water or carbonated water? Does that count?"

Actually, *yes*, fizzy water and seltzer water count! What you *don't* want are the artificially sweetened carbonated waters. Those are a definite no-no. I often crave something fizzy when it's hot outside. So, I always keep a bottle of carbonated water in the fridge.

SPEAKING OF FAUX SUGAR...

Artificial sweeteners are everywhere, and when given the choice between a full-sugar or a "diet" option, chances are, if we are weight-conscious, we'll grab the "diet" or "zero-calorie" choice every time. Why? Psychologically, it sounds like we're doing our body a favor, but we have to look at what these science experiments are doing to our bodies. Plus, we're ingesting chemicals, folks! There's no reason to do that!

Examples of artificial sweeteners are sucralose, aspartame, and saccharin. Three possible things can happen if you consume these chemicals.

You May Crave Sweets

Over time, when you consume artificial sweeteners, the "sweet" taste buds on your tongue are actually dulled down, because artificial sweeteners are so much sweeter than sugar. So, you need more and more sugar and sweetness in your diet to satisfy those cravings. This could lead to overindulging in sweets.

You May Crave Simple Carbs

You could develop cravings for simple carbs like sugar, candy, chips, crackers, cookies, and baked goods. Why? Because the body was tricked into thinking it got some quick energy in the form of sugar. When it realizes it just experienced a chemistry experiment it cannot use, it may crave simple carbs to make up for it and to find that quick energy. If you give in to those cravings, you will begin to gain weight. That is probably not what you intended when you grabbed that "diet" item off the grocery store shelf, right?

The Body May Store the Extra Carbs and Sugar as Fat

Artificial sweeteners can make you crave sugar and simple carbs. Then what? There is no way you can burn all that extra sugar and those carbohydrates without offsetting the calories with extreme physical activity, so if you aren't active enough, your body stores the excess as fat. I remember specifically when I was in college and I started drinking diet sodas. I never knew why, but I was always *starving* after I drank them. Now I know the answer!

There are also many possible negative side effects of artificial sweeteners. Saccharin may cause nausea, diarrhea, skin problems, and other allergy-related issues. It may also be linked to certain cancers. Aspartame may be linked to mood disorders, memory problems, and other neurological illnesses. In some studies, formaldehyde has been found in the livers, kidneys, and brains of test subjects. Sucralose may cause head and muscle aches and is possibly related to multiple sclerosis, stomach cramps, bladder issues, skin irritation, dizziness, and inflammation.

If, like me, you have a serious sweet tooth, you might be wondering, "What's left after you cut out the artificial rubbish?" From my experience, there are more choices than you may think. Do you really want to put those chemicals into your body when there are natural options out there? I think not! You may want to instead try stevia, raw honey, brown rice syrup, or molasses. You can even use applesauce when baking or put it in oatmeal for some natural sweetness. I usually use stevia and raw honey as my natural sweeteners. Stevia is an herb and keeps the blood sugar levels stable. Raw honey is great because it contains many B vitamins and other nutrients. There is also agave nectar, which looks like honey and comes from a cactus. However, there are some new studies that show it may not be as good for us as we think, because it is processed through the liver, which could trigger lipogenesis (a process in which the body produces more fat). So, let's stick with the few that are definitely good.

With so many tasty, all-natural options, there's no reason to keep ingesting the fake stuff. Why load up on chemicals when you don't have to, right? Take a moment to jot down a few items you usually sweeten artificially, and then brainstorm ways you could add sweetness with natural options. To recap, here are some natural sweetener options:

- Stevia
- Raw honey
- Molasses
- Applesauce
- Brown rice syrup

Time to go grocery shopping!

My current artificial sweetener guilty pleasures:

- _____

- _____

- _____

Some natural sweeteners I would like to try:

- _____

- _____

- _____

I'LL HAVE THE SUPER-DUPER-MOCHA FRAPPUCCINO WITH WHIPPED CREAM, PLEASE

Ahhhh, caffeine. One of the ex-loves of my life. We had a really great relationship for many, many years. Then I realized what it was doing to me.

I've been in those coffee shops that are on every corner. It is amazing to me how they are so packed every single morning. People wait in a line that practically stretches out the door for their $4 cup of coffee and they order it like a delicacy on some foreign menu. I've been there, though. I've been that addicted person waiting in line for 10 minutes to get that boost of energy. I've also been the crazy person who took caffeine pills at one point in my life *in addition to drinking coffee*. Then when all those stimulants wore off, I would down energy drinks. Those energy drinks ate holes in my tooth enamel and actually caused several cavities. So again, if this ex-caffeine addict could make progress, so can you.

One coffee drink could have 300, 600, or even 800 calories in it, not to mention 30 to 50 grams of sugar. Add in a scone or muffin and you're off to a carb- and sugar-laden start to your morning, which will only lead you to crash later, crave even more caffeine and sugar, and store fat in the process.

Now, I am not completely anti-caffeine. Here and there is okay. However, it is important to know what it is doing in your body so that you can make your own decision about what is best for you.

The Caffeine/Stimulant Cycle

When a person drinks caffeine or an energy drink, the body feels "stressed," and the fight-or-flight response kicks in. This response was originally designed as a survival mechanism when we had to run from predators and were hunting our food. When a person feels stress from life situations today, the same response occurs. That is why it is so important to reduce stress when trying to lose weight and inches.

When the fight-or-flight response occurs, cortisol, norepinephrine, and epinephrine are released. All the blood rushes *away* from your stomach, your digestive system, your urinary tract, and your reproductive system. Why? You don't need to digest, go to the bathroom, or reproduce when your life is in danger. So immediately, when you feel stress or drink caffeine, your digestion slows down. All the blood rushes to your hands, feet, and brain so you can be alert and "run away" from the stressor.

Cortisol causes weight gain, specifically in the belly area, for several reasons. First, digestion is slowed down. Second, the body increases insulin levels in case we need that extra energy to run from a "predator." Over time, the body becomes resistant to this constant increase in insulin, which could lead to weight gain and type 2 diabetes. Eventually the adrenal glands, which release hormones like cortisol in response to stress, get tired. When this occurs, a person can develop adrenal fatigue.

About 80 percent of American adults experience adrenal fatigue in their lifetime, but it is generally undiagnosed. Symptoms of adrenal fatigue include lethargy and fatigue—especially in the mornings or afternoons—never quite feeling rested even after getting enough sleep, a poor immune system, a decreased libido, increased allergies, muscle or bone loss, depression, and cravings for foods high in salt, sugar, and fat, to name some of the most prominent symptoms. In addition, a person may feel tired from 6:00 p.m. to 9:00 p.m., and then have a sudden energy boost or second wind from 10:00 p.m. to 1:00 a.m.[4]

Now, after reading all these symptoms, you may say, "that's me!" That's what *I* said when I read this, actually. Adrenal fatigue may not show up right away. With me, it was after years and years of not getting enough sleep, drinking energy drinks, living on coffee, and even taking caffeine pills. I did all this in my twenties and it caught up with me in my thirties. Depending on whether you have mild or severe adrenal fatigue, it can take anywhere from six to twenty-four months to completely recover. How do you recover? Drop the caffeine and let those poor adrenal glands rest! The adrenal glands are each about the size of a walnut and one rests on top of each kidney. Poor little guys—they work so hard!

I remember the first time I quit caffeine and stimulants. I had a headache, I felt run down, and I was tired for about two days. On the third day, I started to feel awesome. I have been on and off the caffeine bandwagon a few times, because old habits die hard, but now I am

---

4   James L. Wilson, *Adrenal Fatigue: The 21st Century Stress Syndrome* (Petaluma, CA: Smart Publications, 2001).

officially off. Not only that, but I was recently diagnosed with having a food intolerance to coffee. Who knew that was possible? Needless to say, I am off coffee for good, and I have more energy now than I did when on caffeine. It's funny—I can't even have anything that is "decaf" without getting a slight headache. Why? Because decaf still has a small amount of caffeine in it.

If you have had a coffee habit for a while and drink several cups a day, you may want to wean yourself off slowly. Try to cut out one or two cups, or switch to a half caffeine/half decaf. You may still experience slight headaches, but just know that is the body detoxing itself and that the headaches will pass. I once had a client go from drinking sixteen cups of coffee a day to one cup by weaning himself off slowly. Now that's progress!

Now what? How do we keep our energy up during the day without stimulants? Well, eat something! This is where eating a little something every three hours comes into play. I *always* have food on me, whether it is in my purse or in my car. Nuts, fruit (apples, pears, cherries), veggies, protein bars, almonds, goji berries . . . when you feel that energy crash, it just means your blood sugar levels have dropped. So, rather than reaching for that super-duper-mocha frappaccino with whipped cream, eat from your super-healthy stash of snacks. Your belly fat will also decrease when you quit caffeine. Cool, huh?

WHAT TO DO WHEN LIFE GETS FUN

I love to go out, socialize, and have a beverage or two, but I have noticed that the older I get, the more I feel it the next day! My head hurts, I am *super* bloated, I have no interest in exercising, and I just want to eat garbage. The day after can make me totally regret the fun of the night before—when I'm not planning ahead.

I once went to a Notre Dame football game with my sister. We thought it would be a really good idea to have only hard alcohol and healthy snacks, like fruit, vegetables, and popcorn (to balance out the drinking, of course).

Oh. My. Gosh. I was hurting so much the next day . . . I can't even tell you. Lesson learned! I hardly ever drink hard alcohol now—I stick to mostly wine. When I do drink, I limit it to one or two beverages and make sure I have food on my stomach. Let me share with you a way to go out, enjoy a cocktail or two, and still feel like a normal human being the next day.

Alcohol, in a nutshell, is not the best thing to drink when you're trying to lose inches. First, it tends to lower a person's inhibitions; suddenly a whole pizza or bread basket at the dinner table seems like a really good idea. Alcohol is also a diuretic and will dehydrate you. When trying to lose inches, it is best to limit alcohol to maybe a glass of wine here and there, or eliminate it altogether until you've reached your goal. If you decide to go for it, be sure to count it in your food log so you are not forgetting about the calories you're sipping. Fruity and mixed drinks tend to have the most sugar and calories, so they add up quickly. A frozen margarita can have as many as 250 to 300 calories! Wine is typically about 120 to 150 calories per glass, hard alcohol is about 60 calories per ounce (but be careful what you're mixing it with), and beer is about 120 calories per bottle, unless you get the ultra-light version with only 55 calories. You can also just order a club soda with a twist of lime to stay on your *Lose Your Inches* plan and still have fun. Nobody says you *have* to drink alcohol when in social situations, especially if you are serious about reducing your waistline.

Incidentally, if you do have a few more beverages than you initially planned on and you fear the hangover that may await you the next day, drink coconut water before you go to bed and when you wake up. When a person drinks alcohol, it throws off the potassium-sodium balance in the body; coconut water has six times more potassium than a banana and a bit of sodium as well. Coconut water also helps restore electrolyte balance in the body.

Potassium, sodium, calcium, and magnesium are electrolytes. They help the cells function properly. When you consume alcohol, it makes you dehydrated and depletes these electrolytes, hence, the hangover. That's why it is important to rehydrate and restore those electrolyte levels as soon as possible.

Please note: I am not condoning getting drunk or proposing that drinking coconut water is a miracle cure for hangover. I'm just saying that if you, by chance, had more than you wanted or even if you had just two drinks and feel like a truck ran over you, there is a way to help you feel better faster.

BABY GOALS AND BABY STEPS

During each week of our program, it is important to remember that we are working to build a healthier lifestyle into our daily routine. So let me ask you a few questions:

How much water do you drink each day? _____

What other types of beverages do you usually drink?

_____

_____

_____

How many calories do you consume in your beverages per day?

_____

What are some actions you could implement to drink more water?

_____

_____

_____

Some sample baby goals for this week could be:

1. I will stop getting my grande vanilla latte every day.
2. I will switch to decaf tea or some hot water with lemon for my morning hot beverage.
3. I will reduce my weekly alcohol intake and will record the beverages I drink in my food log.

My three baby goals for this week are:

1. _____

_____

2. _____

_____

3. _____

_____

We've gotten through Week 5. You're doing AWESOME! Think about your journey so far . . . How *proud* are you of yourself? Let's keep going!

Week 5 Measurements

_____Waist (1 in. above belly button)

_____Hips (widest part around glutes)

_____Lower abdomen (2 in. below BB)

_____Right thigh (put right hand flat against leg and measure under the thumb area)

_____Left thigh (put left hand flat against leg and measure under the thumb area)

_____Chest (measure around widest part)

_____Right arm (measure around bicep area)

_____Left arm (measure around bicep area)

_____Right calf (measure around widest part)

_____Left calf (measure around widest part)

_____INCHES LOST THIS WEEK

_____CHANGE SINCE LAST WEEK

_____TOTAL INCHES LOST SO FAR

WEEK 6

Fats, Proteins, and Carbs

How to _Not_ Lose Your Mind: Lesson for Week 6

Fats, proteins, and carbs are actually your friends. You shouldn't have one without the others. It is definitely not a good idea to cut any of the three food groups completely out of your diet. You'll get frustrated, your body won't lose what you want it to lose, and you'll feel terrible. The key is to know how much of each to eat. Then magic happens!

When I first discovered this crazy thing called a food log and counting calories, I noticed right away that just a little portion of food with fat in it had many more calories than foods with little or no fat. For example, a tablespoon of olive oil has 120 calories, and so does an average bowl of cereal. Which would I choose? Hmmm, a spoonful of oil or a whole bowlful of cereal? I immediately became scared of eating fats because I thought that they would _make me fat_! This is some seriously silly thinking, as I'll explain here in a bit.

EATING HEALTHY FATS DOES NOT MAKE YOU FAT

Counting calories without a sense of where they are coming from or where they are going can take you as far off track as not counting them at all. I remember the summer before my second year of college, when I was super gung-ho about losing weight, I thought it would be a fabulous idea to mainly just eat cereal. I would work out for an hour each day (I only did cardio back then—I hadn't yet discovered you always have to include weight training, too), then I would eat 1,200 calories of cereal for the rest of the day—including the milk. I would get those mini-boxes of cereals, so I had quite the variety of sugar cereal deliciousness, and that's what I ate.

I was working out a lot, eating cereal and milk . . . and I didn't lose any weight *or* inches. Why not? Well, basically I was eating all carbs, sugar, and no fat! No healthy fats at all. Without healthy fats, my body was literally *stuck*. The body needs healthy fats to act as lubrication, much like a car engine needs oil to function properly. If there's no oil in the engine, it will fail. Healthy fats act as oil in your body to keep things moving and functioning the way they should.

Interesting side note—people who do not eat enough healthy fats in their diet tend to be constipated more often. Nobody likes to talk about this essential bodily function, but it's true. Healthy fats are also excellent for your hair, skin, nails, brain (obviously an important organ), and for your system overall. They even can help raise HDL cholesterol, which is the "good" cholesterol. It may seem counter-productive to eat healthy fats, but if you want to lose fat, you need incorporate them into your diet. Pure and simple.

TYPES OF FATS

There are basically three types of fats: trans, saturated, and unsaturated. What's the difference?

Trans: Most people know by now that these are the killer fats. Trans fats are man-made in a chemical lab and can clog the arteries, leading to heart attacks and strokes. Make sure that the foods you eat do not contain hydrogenated or partially hydrogenated oils, because these are trans fats. Examples of foods that contain trans fats are margarine, shortening, fast food, french fries, baked goods like donuts, muffins, and cookies, fried foods, chips, crackers, candy, dips, salad dressings, packaged foods, and even some frozen foods and soups. Just look at the label and make sure it says "0 trans fat."

Saturated: These are fats that are solid at room temperature. Ideally, you want to have less than 10 percent of your daily calories from saturated fat. It used to be thought that all saturated fats were bad. However, there are studies now that show some, like coconut oil, provide health benefits.

Foods that contain saturated fats I would stay away from or limit include processed or packaged foods, candy, baked goods, sausage, bacon, cookies, whipped cream, crackers, fast food, and fatty meat. One question I get sometimes is, "Which is better—butter or margarine?" I would actually recommend using real butter in small amounts versus margarine, because, well, margarine contains trans fats. Be mindful when you are grocery shopping, and read the labels.

Unsaturated: These are healthy fats that are found in foods like olive oil, nuts, seeds, and avocados. There are two types of unsaturated fats—*monounsaturated* and *polyunsaturated*. "Mono" means that there is one double-bonded unsaturated carbon in the molecule. "Poly" means there are many double-bonded unsaturated carbons in the molecule.

Examples of monounsaturated fats are olive oil, peanut oil, sesame oil, peanut butter, almond butter, avocados, macadamia nuts, pecans, hazelnuts, almonds, olives, and seeds.

Examples of polyunsaturated fats are walnuts, sunflower seeds, grapeseed oil, safflower oil, salmon, herring, and trout. Omega-3 fatty acids are super healthy for you and also fall under this category. Omega-3s are made up of three fatty acids—ALA (alpha-lipoic acid), EPA (eicosapentaenoic acid), and DHA (docosahexaenoic acid). You don't have to remember the scientific names—just remember that omega-3s are very healthy for you.

Omega-3s help reduce inflammation; are great for the brain, skin, and nails; help reduce anxiety, stress, and depression; and can be beneficial for those with ADD or ADHD. These healthy fats also increase HDL (the good cholesterol) and lower LDL (the bad cholesterol). We want our HDL to be high, because it helps remove the LDL from our bodies. Omega-3s can be found in fish oil, cod liver oil, krill oil, and in fatty fish like salmon. They can also be found in foods like walnuts, almonds, sardines, and chia seeds.

In choosing between taking a fish oil supplement versus flaxseed oil,

I would choose the fish oil supplement. Why? Because the body is not as efficient in breaking down the ALA in flaxseed oil and converting it to omega-3s. So, it's more efficient just to take fish oil, because the body does not have to convert it and you can be sure you'll get your omega-3s. Plus, fish oil contains EPA and DHA, but flaxseed oil does not. EPA and DHA offer many health benefits, especially for heart health.

To summarize what we just learned, trans fats can clog the arteries, saturated fats should be less than 10 percent of your diet, and monounsaturated and polyunsaturated fats are healthy fats to incorporate into your daily eating plan.

For your reference, here is a list of fats to avoid:

Fats to Avoid or Limit in Your Diet

Baked goods (cookies, muffins, croissants, donuts, scones, pastries, cakes)

Shortening

Margarine

Salad dressings

Prepackaged desserts

Frozen meals

Chips

Crackers

Bacon

Sausage

Fast food

French fries

All fried foods

Dips

Candy bars

Healthy Fats to Include in Your Diet

Avocados

Olive oil

Coconut oil

Almonds

Walnuts

Brazil nuts

Pistachios

Macadamia nuts

Pecans

Hazelnuts

Olives

Organic peanut butter, almond butter, or cashew butter

Omega-3 fatty acids such as in fish oil, cod liver oil, or krill oil

Fatty fish like wild Alaskan salmon, sockeye salmon, herring, or freshwater trout

Sardines

Seeds like sunflower or chia seeds

Peanut oil

Sesame oil

Grapeseed oil

HOW TO INCORPORATE HEALTHY FATS INTO YOUR DIET

I want to expand a little more on healthy fats and how to enjoy them in our daily diet. As I mentioned earlier, avocados are wonderful for you, one of the best healthy fats ever. If you have low HDL or high LDL, try eating half an avocado a day. You can just slice it up and eat it or mash it to make some fresh guacamole.

As far as oils go, olive oil is probably the best vegetable oil for us. I use regular olive oil for cooking and extra virgin olive oil when I am making salad dressings and other dishes where the taste is important enough to justify the added expense.

Another oil you might like to try (especially if you have low thyroid function) is coconut oil. You can cook with it, put it in oatmeal or anything hot, or put it in a smoothie. You can even use it directly on your skin as a moisturizer! Coconut oil has a lot of other added benefits, and it can also help speed up your metabolism. I love to reference a study that was done in the 1940s.[5] A group of farmers decided to add coconut oil to the cattle feed, hoping to fatten up their stock. However, the cows became skinny (who wants a skinny cow?) and they had more energy than before. Then the farmers decided to add soy and corn to the cattle feed, and they became fat. Soy and corn has been a staple in livestock feed ever since.

Why would coconut oil make the cows skinny? The reason is that coconut oil is a medium-chain fatty acid that quickly converts to energy and is not stored in the body as fat or cholesterol. There are many ways to incorporate coconut oil into your diet. For those who have hypothyroidism—low thyroid function—you *must* look up online the benefits of coconut oil for the thyroid. There are also several books completely dedicated to the benefits of coconut oil. You will be amazed!

Do you love peanut butter? I *love* peanut butter! Go with a natural or organic peanut butter. There are stir and no-stir brands, so you can find one that doesn't have the oil floating on top. Or, you can try almond butter, which is also delicious—it's just like peanut butter but with a slightly nuttier taste. In the health food store and in some grocery stores, you can actually make your own peanut butter! There is a machine that just crushes a bunch of peanuts. That's what I use—

---

5 Raymond Peat, "Coconut Oil," available at http://coconutoil.com/ray_peat_coconutoil/

I love it. You can even make your own peanut butter or almond butter with a food processor. Talk about minimal ingredients and knowing exactly what's in what you just made!

I just want to take a moment to talk a little bit more about omega-3s. These are by far the *best* fats for you. Omega-3 supplements are made from fish, krill, and cod liver oil. Omega-3s are a natural anti-inflammatory agent, so if you have arthritis, joint pain, or are just inflamed from other health issues, you need omega-3s. I've had clients who substantially reduced their arthritis symptoms simply by taking omega-3s every day. The minimum recommended dose on the label is about 1,000 mg per day. Some people can take more, depending on their health condition, but *consult your doctor first.*

The key to getting the benefits of omega-3s is to buy the *right kind*! When buying fish oil, make sure the label says "pharmaceutical grade" and "molecularly distilled." You also want it to say "no mercury, toxins, or PCBs." PCB stands for "polychlorinated biphenyls," which are manufactured chemicals and may be carcinogens. Mercury is a heavy metal that can actually attach to your organs and make them slowly shut down, which is what happens with mercury poisoning. The type of mercury found in fish is called methylmercury. Early signs of mercury poisoning are headaches, fatigue, and impaired cognitive ability. Symptoms increase as toxicity increases. Signs of severe toxicity could include muscle pain, indigestion, tremors, insomnia, constipation, anemia, dizziness, poor coordination, pins-and-needles feelings in the hands and feet, and difficulties with walking, hearing, and speech.[6] Even the EPA has recognized that fetal exposure to methylmercury can adversely affect the baby's developing brain and nervous system.

The best types of salmon are wild Alaskan salmon and sockeye salmon. They contain the lowest amounts of mercury and are super high in omega-3s. You can also find this type of salmon canned. In general, the smaller the fish, the less mercury it contains. The reason is

6   Michael T. Murray and Joseph Pizzorno, *The Encyclopedia of Natural Medicine*, 3rd ed. (New York: Atria, 2012), 110–11.

because bigger fish eat smaller fish: The higher up the food chain, the heavier the concentration of mercury.

Here is a list of which fish are high and low in mercury according to the US Food and Drug Administration. The fish are listed in order from lowest (scallops) to highest (tilefish) in the average amount of mercury concentration:

Fish Lowest in Mercury

Scallops (the lowest in mercury)

Salmon (canned)

Clams

Shrimp

Oysters

Sardines

Tilapia

Anchovies

Salmon (fresh or frozen—wild Alaskan and sockeye are best)

Squid (calamari)

Catfish

Pollock

Crawfish

Atlantic mackerel

Mullet

Whiting

Atlantic haddock

Flatfish (Flounder, Plaice, Sole)

Butterfish

Crab (Blue, King, Snow)

Atlantic croaker

Freshwater trout

Hake

Jacksmelt

Herring

Pacific mackerel chub

Ocean perch

Fish Low in Mercury
(no more than six 6-oz. servings per month)

Lobster (spiny)

Carp

Alaskan cod

Skate

Skipjack tuna	Mahi Mahi
Freshwater perch	Scorpionfish
Bass (Striped, Black, Rockfish)	Weakfish (sea trout)
Snapper	Halibut
Monkfish	Pacific white croaker
Spanish mackerel (S. Atlantic)	Canned, chunk light tuna

Fish High in Mercury
(no more than three 6-oz. servings per month)

Albacore tuna	Bluefish
Chilean sea bass	Grouper
Yellowfin tuna	Spanish mackerel (Gulf of Mexico)
Sablefish	

Fish Highest in Mercury *(avoid eating)*

Marlin	Shark
Orange roughy	Swordfish
Ahi and bigeye tuna	Tilefish (Gulf of Mexico—the highest in mercury)
King mackerel	

Now that you know which fish are high and low in mercury, you can make smarter choices when grocery shopping or dining out. I think most people should take an omega-3 supplement every day since many people do not eat enough fatty fish in their diet. I certainly take my omega-3s daily. They come in gel cap or liquid form. If you take the liquid version, just put it in a little freshly made juice and enjoy! You won't even taste it. Omega-3s can also help those with anxiety, depression, and stress, and can even help kids with ADD or ADHD.

HOW MUCH FAT SHOULD BE IN MY DIET?

Now with all fats, even healthy ones, you need to watch the portions. If you eat nuts, look at the label and try to stick to that one-quarter-cup serving size, which is usually anywhere from twenty to twenty-five pieces. If you use olive oil, read the label and try to stick to a tablespoon or two. With peanut butter, as much as I love it and could eat the whole jar (which I once did in college—don't ask—my tummy was *really* hurting the next day), you have to measure it. Eat 1 to 2 tablespoons maximum for the day, because each tablespoon is about 95 calories.

Overall, as healthy and as necessary as these healthy fats are to your eating plan, you do have to pay attention, because you can over-indulge, just as with any other food. The USDA states that we should have between 20 percent and 35 percent of our daily calories from fat. Each gram of fat contains 9 calories, so, if you're eating 1,800 calories a day, for example, then you could eat 360–630 calories from fat. A sample daily consumption of fat might look like this: 2 tbsp. peanut butter (190 cal.), 2 tbsp. olive oil (240 cal.), 1 tbsp. coconut oil (117 cal.), and about ten almonds (70 cal.) That totals to 617 calories from fat. Obviously, if you eat less than 1,800 calories a day, your numbers will be different.

WANT TO LOOK TONED? EAT PROTEIN!

Every man and woman says the same thing: "I want to be toned." On the other hand, nobody says, "I want to be bulky or skinny with no muscle tone." One preconceived notion I hope we have thrown out the window by now is that weight training will bulk you up. To really look as bulky as a weightlifter, you have to do a lot of interesting things with diet and supplements—things that the average person has no interest in.

With resistance training and exercise, the body literally breaks down muscle then builds it back up again to make it even stronger than before. This is how you get a toned look. Muscle is made of protein, and the building blocks of protein are amino acids. If you don't eat enough protein, you could lift weights for many hours a day and you still will *not* get that toned look you want. It's a pretty basic equation:

Protein = muscle, and muscle = toning.

Now, which foods have protein? Eggs are one of my favorites—cheap, easy to cook, and good for you. If possible, only buy free-range or organic eggs. Each whole egg has 6 grams of protein, and each egg white by itself has 4 grams of protein. So, you can use two eggs or a few egg whites and make a quick omelet to get about 12 to 18 grams of protein in one meal.

Other good sources of protein are chicken, turkey, lean beef, fish, beans, and nuts. Protein bars and protein shakes are always a great addition to any diet, but read the labels and be sure to buy the more natural or organic brands, without all those chemicals and artificial sweeteners. A protein bar can have 10 to 30 grams of protein, and a scoop of protein powder could have 15 to 30 grams of protein as well.

My vegan and vegetarian friends have more of a challenge in getting adequate protein in their diet. Legumes are going to be your best friend if you don't eat eggs or fish. A cup of lentils, for example, has about 18 grams of protein. Kidney, black, and pinto beans also have about 18 grams of protein per cup. Beans and rice together also make a complete protein combination, as all of the essential amino acids are present when these two foods are eaten together.

A great whole grain that is also a complete protein is quinoa (pronounced *keen-wah*). Quinoa contains 15 percent protein, so you get 8 grams of protein per cup of cooked quinoa, whereas brown rice only has 5 grams of protein per cup.

HOW MUCH PROTEIN SHOULD BE IN MY DIET?

How much protein should you actually be consuming? The USDA says that adults should have 10–35 percent of their daily calories from protein. One gram of protein equals 4 calories. Here are some simple formulas to figure out what your daily protein intake should be.

The RDA (Recommended Daily Allowance) guideline for *minimum* protein intake for adults is *0.8 g protein/kg of body weight or 0.36 g protein/lb. of body weight.* To find the minimum amount of protein you should be eating, take your body weight and multiply it by 0.36.

For example, a person weighing 150 pounds should consume at least 54 grams of protein per day.

$$150 \text{ lbs.} \times 0.36 = 54 \text{ g protein}$$

If a person is a weightlifter, bodybuilder, or athlete, then the protein recommendations increase. The International Society of Sports Nutrition recommends 0.73–0.96 grams of protein per pound of body weight for these athletes. Here is an example of how to calculate that range for a 150-pound person:

$$150 \text{ lbs.} \times 0.73 = 109.5 \text{ g protein}$$
$$150 \text{ lbs.} \times 0.96 = 144 \text{ g protein}$$

So, a typical 150-pound adult should eat a minimum of 54 grams of protein per day. If the individual is a bodybuilder, weightlifter, or athlete who is very physically active, he or she can have between 109.5 and 144 grams of protein per day.

I always recommend that a person eat at *least* the recommended 0.36 grams of protein per pound of body weight. So, in our example here, that person should eat at least 54 grams of protein per day. Should you ever go under your minimum? Absolutely not! Can you go over your protein range? Sure. I always eat above my minimum. Protein just makes me feel good and keeps me fuller longer. Plus, I work out five days a week, combining both cardio and strength training. You'll know if you are getting the right amount of protein by how you feel. In general, most people I coach seem to eat too little protein. If you are eating too little protein, you may then crave sweets and simple carbs such as candy, cookies, chips, bread, or crackers, so pay attention to your cravings. These cravings result because your body is trying to find some quick energy. Protein breaks down slowly in the body when we eat it and helps keep our blood sugar levels stable.

As I mentioned earlier, some body builders will eat 0.73–0.96 grams of protein per pound of bodyweight. They are going for a specific goal of muscle gain. However, they are also lifting heavy weights, breaking down those muscles, and building them back up again. This much protein may be too hard on the system for some people, but everyone is different. Low-carb diets, in my opinion, require too much protein and fat. Our liver then has to process it all. If a person eats too much protein, just as if too many carbs or too much fat is consumed, it can result in weight gain if the extra calories are not burned.

So, how much protein are you eating currently? Here are some examples of common food items and their protein content. See other examples of proteins on page 88. You can also look up other items on your handy internet calorie counter, phone app, or calorie-counter booklet.

Food	Protein
1 egg	6 g
1 egg white	4 g
3 oz. chicken breast	24 g
3 oz. lean beef	23 g
3 oz. fish	18 g
1 cup legumes (beans)	15 g
1 cup quinoa	8 g
1 cup plain Greek yogurt	14 g
1 string cheese	6 g
1 oz. almonds (23 nuts)	6 g

My weight in pounds _____ × 0.36 =

_____ My minimum grams of protein per day

How much protein I am eating now:

_____

How much protein I need to eat per day at a minimum:

_____

Which foods can I incorporate more into my diet to meet my goal amount of protein?

Food	Grams of Protein
1.	
2.	
3.	
4.	
5.	
Total Grams of Protein	

CARBOHYDRATES

The dietary guideline for Americans by the US Department of Agriculture states that 45–65 percent of our diet should come from carbohydrates. One gram of carbohydrates equals 4 calories. No, this doesn't mean chips, crackers, bread, and cookies. It means those unprocessed, natural carbohydrates like fruits, vegetables, oats, beans, rice, quinoa, and everything in between. I always say the closer you eat to what God naturally put on Earth, the better.

Another point to think about is that carbs are not the enemy. When the low-carb craze started, people immediately became scared to eat any carbs. I once tried the low-carb diet for an entire summer, and I felt *terrible*—I had no energy, my brain was foggy, and I had this weird, metallic taste in my mouth. To this day, we still think all carbs are bad! However, we need them for energy. When we eat carbohydrates, they break down into something called glucose. Glucose is actually *what our brains run on*, so we need carbs! If you've ever tried one of those low-carb diets, chances are you felt lethargic, had brain fog, and were just out of it. Why? Because you didn't have enough carbohydrates to produce the glucose you needed. You were functioning on ketones, or "fat cells." This initially may seem like a good idea. However, this is a back-up mechanism developed by the body to keep us safe from starvation. So, if you lived during the hunter-gatherer period of time and you didn't catch your food that day, burning fat cells meant you could live a little longer. But this is not a sustainable way to live, and your body doesn't like it for long periods of time. Carbs are our *friends*! We just need to eat the right ones.

In that spirit, let's have a little carbohydrate education. There are two types of carbs: simple and complex. The difference between the two is the rate of digestion and absorption in the body.

Simple Carbs

These are carbs that break down quickly in the body and convert to glucose. Simple carbs are made of a single sugar unit of glucose, fructose, and galactose.[7] Simple carbs can occur naturally, such as in fruit, or in processed foods, such as in candy bars, doughnuts, bagels, and cookies. Overall, you want to limit your simple carb intake, because it raises your blood sugar levels and causes your body to secrete insulin. Over time, the pancreas could work too hard if you have too much sugar in your diet, leading to diabetes, because your body becomes insulin-resistant. So, only eat simple carbs that are natural, like those found in fruit, because they have fiber and nutrients, which help them break down more slowly.

Complex Carbs

These are carbs that are starches and made of long chains of glucose.[8] Some examples of these are vegetables, sweet potatoes, yams, wholegrain cereals, quinoa, rice, oats, and legumes. Complex carbs digest

---

7   Staci Nix, *Williams' Basic Nutrition and Diet Therapy*, 13th ed. (St. Louis: Mosby Elsevier, 2009), 14–17.

8   Ibid.

slower in the body, causing the body to release less insulin and not caus-ing the blood sugar to spike as much, so you don't get that roller coaster effect. This creates a constant energy level rather than the highs and lows of simple carbs. The same rule applies, though: Get your complex carbs from natural sources, not processed.

You will know how many carbs your body needs based on how you *feel*. If you wake up bloated one day, then you probably had too many carbs the day before (or sodium or alcohol). The term "hydrate" in the word "carbohydrate" literally means water, so carbs naturally con-tain water. The more carbs you eat that aren't natural, the more water you'll retain.

You also need to pay attention to how you *feel* when you eat certain carbs. I know that if I eat rice, my stomach will be bloated and gaseous later on. It's just how my body reacts to rice. Potatoes, sweet or regular, agree with my system. I can handle oatmeal in small amounts, and a little pasta if it's brown-rice pasta. I can handle most fruits, but some of them make me hungry. So, just pay attention to how your body feels. The next time you eat potatoes, rice, pasta, or even fruit, notice how long you stay full and how your system reacts. You may also want to write on your food log how you feel after eating certain carbs.

BABY GOALS AND BABY STEPS

Looking back over what we learned about fats, proteins, and carbohy-drates, let's start moving forward with three baby goals—one for each category.

Some sample baby goals for this week could be:

1. I will actually buy an avocado and cut it open at home . . . then eat it.
2. I will blend a new shake with frozen fruit, almond milk, and protein powder.
3. I will cook some brown rice pasta, or quinoa.

So, what's going to work for you?

My three baby goals for this week are:

1. _____

  _____

2. _____

  _____

3. _____

  _____

Fantastic! Now it is time to take our measurements again—isn't it funny how it gets easier and easier to check your inches when you've been giving your body the right nutrients in the right amounts?

Week 6 Measurements

_____Waist (1 in. above belly button)

_____Hips (widest part around glutes)

_____Lower abdomen (2 in. below BB)

_____Right thigh (put right hand flat against leg and measure under the thumb area)

_____Left thigh (put left hand flat against leg and measure under the thumb area)

_____Chest (measure around widest part)

_____Right arm (measure around bicep area)

_____Left arm (measure around bicep area)

_____Right calf (measure around widest part)

_____Left calf (measure around widest part)

_____INCHES LOST THIS WEEK

_____CHANGE SINCE LAST WEEK

_____TOTAL INCHES LOST SO FAR

WEEK 7

Fitness

WHY YOU HAVE TO EXERCISE

Are you tired of hearing about exercise yet? No? Good, because I'm not done talking about it!

The body isn't meant to sit all day. Since the beginning of time, humans have had to hunt, run, plant, haul, fetch water, build houses, and make clothing and tools. The body is an incredible machine that is designed to be active. These days, most people work indoors in front of a computer all day—the exact opposite of what the body is designed to do. When the body exercises, it is happy to be useful, which is then reflected in your overall health and in your waistline. Our bodies are made to move, and our muscles are made to be used.

Exercise is important for lowering blood pressure, lowering LDL (bad) cholesterol, improving HDL (good) cholesterol, improving blood glucose levels, and preventing diabetes. It can even help *reverse* type 2 diabetes, and it certainly improves your heart health. Not only that, but you feel good after you exercise. The brain releases these awesome neurotransmitters called endorphins that keep a person coming back for more. Exercise boosts your endorphins, which makes you feel good, and when you feel good, you start to naturally make better choices about everything . . . including food.

WHY DO YOU LIKE EXERCISE? WHY DID YOU STOP EXERCISING IN THE PAST?

Way back in Week 4 (I'm kidding, it really wasn't that long ago) we first introduced exercise in our campaign to lose your inches. We spoke about two kinds of exercise: cardiovascular exercise, or cardio, and strength/resistance training. Did you take up the challenge to begin exercising in Week 4? Did you increase and augment your exercise program? Did you join a gym or at least visit one to see what kind of programs they offer? Did you work out with a friend or your significant other? Did you meet with a personal trainer? Did you head out the door for a 10-minute walk? What did you do that you liked?

What I want you to do now is to write down five things about exercise that you now enjoy. It could be something like

1. I love running.
2. I like working out in the mornings.
3. I like the way exercise breaks up my day.
4. I like not having to think about anything while I exercise.
5. I love exercising outdoors and getting some fresh air.

My top 5 favorite things about exercise are:

1. _____

   _____

2. _____

   _____

3. _____

_____

4. _____

_____

5. _____

_____

Now that you've noticed your five favorite things about exercise, do you see a pattern? Are you a gym person? A class person? A workout-on-your-own person? An early-morning-before-the-kids-wake-up person? An outdoor person?

Since you now know what you enjoy about exercise, let's figure out why you may have stopped exercising in the past, if you did. The reason is that I want you to keep exercising, even after these ten weeks are over.

Please note: If you have kept up your exercise routine, then you can answer the next set of questions from the perspective of, "What keeps me from exercising as much as I would like?"

Here are some common excuses you may have used in the past:

I had no time.

I lost motivation.

I got bored.

I changed jobs.

I moved.

I got married/got into a new relationship.

I didn't see results fast enough.

It got cold outside.

I stopped putting myself first.

I got lazy.

You get the picture. Write down up to five reasons that made you stop or reduce your ideal exercise in the past:

The top 5 reasons I stopped exercising/didn't exercise as much as I wanted to are:

1. _____

   _____

2. _____

   _____

3. _____

   _____

4. _____

   _____

5. _____

   _____

Most people fall off the exercise bandwagon after a week or two. If you have stopped exercising completely or are exercising less than you would like since you designed a program for yourself a few weeks ago, have you noticed changes in your lifestyle? Some things that may have happened when you stopped exercising or reduced your exercise are

I put on weight.

I started eating junk foods.

I started craving sweets.

I stopped caring about how I look.

I feel more depressed.

My blood pressure increased.

I don't sleep very well.

I have no energy.

I feel drained all the time.

This list could go on forever, which should show you just *how important* exercise is. Go ahead, make your list.

Note: Even if you are exercising regularly, make this list based on a time when you had to skip several days in a row, perhaps because of a vacation, holiday, or busy time at work—it's a great thing to keep in the forefront of your mind!

When I stopped exercising or reduced the amount of exercise I would like to do each day, I noticed that the following happened:

1. _____

   _____

2. _____

   _____

3. _____

   _____

4. _____

   _____

5. _____

   _____

HOW MUCH CARDIO SHOULD I BE DOING?

In Week 4 we talked about how you have to do both types of exercise—cardio and resistance training (weight training) to get the results you want. You do not want to only do cardio, because this can result in the skinny-fat person with no muscle tone. The perfect workout consists of resistance training exercises that also raise your heart rate so you can get both cardio *and* resistance training at the exact same time. Efficient, eh?

It is important to do cardiovascular exercise each week. Raising your heart rate, ideally for 30 minutes, three to five times a week, has tremendous benefits for both your long-term health and your short-term happiness.

Here are some examples of cardio exercises:

Running	Elliptical	Zumba®
Walking	Dancing	Kickboxing
Swimming	Jumping rope	Boxing
Jogging	Aerobics classes	Stair climbing
Cycling	Skiing	Rowing

All of these activities will elevate your heart rate if performed at the appropriate intensity. Just taking a stroll or doing housework doesn't count. For example, an hour of walking at a brisk pace burns about 351 calories for a 150-pound adult. On the other hand, vacuuming and doing other light household work like dusting and cleaning for an hour only burns 198 calories.

It is important to enjoy the cardio exercise or exercises you choose. If you enjoy what you do, you will stick with it . . . are you sensing a theme here?

There is something called the "talk test" that helps you measure if you are getting your heart rate up high enough during exercise. The talk test is as simple as this:

Too Easy: If you can easily carry on a conversation while exercising, you're not working hard enough.

Moderate: If you are slightly winded while exercising and can still carry on a conversation, even if it's a bit labored, you are at a good intensity.

Too Hard: If you are gasping for air and cannot carry on a conversation at all, let alone catch your breath, you are working too hard and need to slow down.

You want to stay in the "moderate" range—slightly winded, yet still able to carry on a conversation.

HOW MUCH RESISTANCE TRAINING SHOULD I BE DOING?

Resistance training, or weight training, will help a person lose weight, lose inches, increase bone strength, help prevent osteoporosis, and help boost the metabolism by increasing muscle mass so that you burn more calories all day long—even while watching television. Studies have shown that up to two hours after a cardio session, exercisers will burn more calories than if they had completed no workout. However, after a resistance training session, a person can burn extra calories for *up to thirty-eight hours.*[9] Nice!

Resistance training also reshapes the body. Cardio may shrink the body, but it will *not* reshape it the way you envision. You will keep the same shape, just smaller. If you want those abs to finally show up, have a flat stomach, lift those sagging glutes, and lose the chicken wings under the arms, you have to do resistance training.

There are seven major muscle groups: chest, back, shoulders, biceps, triceps, abdominals, and legs. The largest muscle groups will ultimately burn the most calories throughout the day, so those are the ones we

9   M. D. Schuenke, R. P. Mikat, and J. M. McBride, "Effect of an Acute Period of Resistance Exercise on Excess Post-Exercise Oxygen Consumption: Implications for Body Mass Management," *European Journal of Applied Physiology* 86, no. 5 (March 2002): 411–7, doi:10.1007/s00421-001-0568-y. PMID 11882927.

want to be sure to work out often. The largest muscle groups are the legs and lower body. The next largest are the chest and back, then the abdominals and shoulders, and the smallest are the biceps and triceps.

The next thing to know is that each muscle group has a counterpart. For example, the biceps and the triceps are opposite muscle groups that work together. Think about when you lift a bottle of water off your desk to drink it. When you lift it up, you are engaging your bicep (the front of your arms) and the tricep (back of your arm) is relaxing. When you put the bottle back down, the bicep is now relaxing and the tricep is engaged.

Other opposing muscle groups are chest and back, quads and hamstrings, and abs and lower back. So, when you work one muscle group, you have to be sure to work the opposing muscle group. For example, you don't want to just work your chest and have huge chest muscles, but then forget about your upper back. This could cause posture problems and injury in the long run. Likewise, you don't want to work just abs and forget about the lower back. Having strong abs and a weak back is a great way to strain the lower back.

Ideally, you want to work each major muscle group during every workout. Concentrate on full-body movements, because (1) it is the most efficient way to work out, and (2) you don't want to work out forever! Why spend two hours in a gym slowly working each muscle group individually when you can combine them and be done in 30 minutes? See my logic?

If you are just starting out with resistance training, it is a good idea to begin with your gym's basic circuit of weight machines. Usually the gym will have the machines in an order that allows you to work each body part. Over time, advance slowly by increasing either the amount of weight or the number of reps on each exercise.

There are two basic concepts you need to learn with regards to weight training:

Rep: A "rep" is short for repetition. For example, on one exercise, you may do ten to fifteen repetitions, meaning you are repeating the same movement over and over. If I am doing a bicep curl fifteen times, then that is fifteen reps.

Set: A "set" is a grouping of a number of reps. You should do two to three sets of most exercises. For example, if I just completed my fifteen bicep curls, that is set 1. If I completed another fifteen reps after resting for a few minutes, that is set 2. One more set of fifteen after that would be set 3. Simple, right?

To figure out the number of reps you should be doing for each exercise, aim for the last two or three reps to be difficult; you should struggle to complete them. I suggest doing three sets of ten to twelve reps per exercise. If your last two or three reps are challenging and you feel the burn, you are at a correct weight amount. On the other hand, if you do fifteen bicep curls and feel you can do ten more, then the weight isn't heavy enough. You want to keep the weight heavy enough so the muscles will grow and you'll achieve a toned look.

If you are designing your own weights routine, choose eight to ten of your favorite exercises that work each body part. Here is a sample full-body routine:

1. 12 regular squats (legs)
2. 12 dumbbell rows, each side (upper back)
3. 12 bicep curls (arms)
4. 12 tricep dips (arms)
5. 12 shoulder presses (shoulders)
6. 12 standing lunges—left leg in front
7. 12 standing lunges—right leg in front
8. 12 push-ups—regular or knee (chest)
9. 12 Supermans (lower back)
10. 12 full sit-ups (abs)

Repeat entire sequence two or three times for a full workout.

As you can see here, these exercises have worked *all* of the major muscle groups. I can follow these exercises in order and do twelve reps of each and two or three sets total. You would do a full-body workout like this one every *other* day, not two days in a row. So, Monday, Wednesday, and Friday could be "weights" days, and then Tuesday and Thursday would be cardio days. Saturday could also be a light cardio day or rest day, and then Sunday you rest.

DON'T FORGET!

All this talk about exercise and reps and heart rate is very valuable, but we don't want to lose track of our regular activity throughout the day, either. In other words, sitting at a desk for eight hours and going to the gym for a half hour or 45 minutes is great, but we also want to pay attention to opportunities that may arise in our daily life to increase our activity level, burn more calories, and raise our overall metabolism.

For example:

Can you walk up the stairs at your office or apartment instead of taking the elevator?

Can you walk to do your errands, instead of driving? Or drive somewhere central and walk to your various locations from there? (Extra credit if you actually carry something heavy, like groceries, back to your car on your walk.)

Can you choose a family activity like a hike instead of going out to eat?

Can you walk your dog beyond the least amount of time required for Poncho or Bubbles to "take care of business"?

Can you rake your own leaves into a pile instead of using a leaf blower?

Can you park at the end of the parking lot when going to the store, so you have to walk farther? (I *always* do this, plus it helps protect your car from dings!)

Can you go outside and throw the ball with your kids?

Can you walk your kids to their friend's house that is a minute drive away, instead of taking the car?

BABY GOALS AND BABY STEPS

Exercise, like everything else, requires a little bit of planning and a little bit of foresight. We implemented exercise in Week 4. You've had three weeks to get exercise into your life. If you find now that your exercise routine needs a little fine-tuning or adjusting, this is the week to do so. Again, we are going for lifestyle changes here.

If you have decided over the past few weeks that you are an exercise class person but haven't loved the classes you've tried, you may have to research new classes in your local area. If you have decided you are an outside workout person, are you getting outside as often as you like? Do you need to join a running group or an outdoor boot camp to keep you motivated? If you had wanted to work out with a friend or significant other but that never quite panned out, maybe it's time to readjust and do things on your own. A lifestyle of exercise requires planning. You can start and continue with baby steps.

Some sample baby goals for this week could be:

1. I will use the "Talk Test" next time I work out to make sure I am exercising at a good enough intensity.
2. I will try the weights circuit in my gym.
3. I will try that Zumba® class my friends have been telling me about.

My three baby goals for this week are:

1. _____

_____

2. _____

_____

3. _____

_____

Seven weeks down and three to go. We're almost there! Those jeans are going to look *great* on you!

Week 7 Measurements

_____ Waist (1 in. above belly button)

_____ Hips (widest part around glutes)

_____ Lower abdomen (2 in. below BB)

_____ Right thigh (put right hand flat against leg and measure under the thumb area)

_____ Left thigh (put left hand flat against leg and measure under the thumb area)

_____ Chest (measure around widest part)

_____ Right arm (measure around bicep area)

_____ Left arm (measure around bicep area)

_____ Right calf (measure around widest part)

_____ Left calf (measure around widest part)

_____ INCHES LOST THIS WEEK

_____ CHANGE SINCE LAST WEEK

_____ TOTAL INCHES LOST SO FAR

WEEK 8

Cravings, Bingeing, and Other Foes of Losing Your Inches

> **How to *Not* Lose Your Mind: Lesson for Week 8**
>
> Here's the deal: We all have cravings. Those cravings simply mean that *our body is trying to talk to us*. The trick is to figure out what it is saying!

In Week 3, we talked about what happens when we have been "good" all day (i.e., we barely ate all day) . . . and then we lose control at dinnertime, during dessert, or in the middle of the night. I actually know someone who was injured while tripping down the stairs, trying to get to a midnight snack—not funny to them at the time, but a good reminder to us all (was this you?). Calorie counting never rests. Remember, your target caloric intake is for an entire twenty-four-hour period. So what throws us off track? Three things, really: cravings, mindless eating, and speed eating. Let's take a look at each of these in more detail.

THE CAUSE BEHIND CRAVINGS

Our body's most common cravings are sugar, salt, caffeine, and alcohol. In my work with women, cravings for sweets seem to be more prevalent. Alcohol and caffeine cravings seem to be pretty gender neutral. Men seem to crave more greasy and salty foods. Of course, everybody is different. The big question is, what causes these cravings, and what do they mean?

Cravings mean that your body is lacking something, either a certain nutrient, a mineral, or even something as simple as sleep. Some cravings can also be caused by external factors, like stress, anxiety, lone-liness, or plain old boredom. Let's get a little more specific about why cravings occur. As you read this list, pay attention to whether any of these items relate to you:

A Craving Can Occur If . . .

You wait too long to eat between meals.

You don't eat enough during the day.

You didn't get enough sleep.

You skip breakfast.

You don't eat enough protein.

You don't get enough sweet-tasting foods from natural sources, such as fruits or sweet-tasting vegetables like sweet potatoes.

You are lonely or lacking in emotional sweetness.

You are dehydrated and need to drink more water.

You rarely eat healthy fats.

Your meals typically lack color—e.g., fruits or vegetables.

You drink a lot of caffeine, sodas, or sugary drinks.

Your meals are typically high in sodium.

Have you ever eaten something super sweet and then instantly craved something salty afterward? Have you ever eaten a meal that is heavy in meat or salt, and then instantly craved something sweet after-ward? That craving occurs because your body is trying to create some balance. Realizing this yin and yang relationship is good practice to learn what your body is telling you. Salty and sweet are one example of extremes. Hot and cold are another extreme. Smooth and crunchy are yet another extreme. I know that if I have a smoothie, I actually will crave something crunchy right after. If you have too much of one extreme, you will often crave the other extreme, which is why it makes sense that the best way to combat cravings is to have *balance* in your diet.

Balancing foods are fruits; vegetables; whole grains; dark, leafy greens; beans; and legumes. So, have your sweet and salty foods, but be sure to incorporate those balanced foods into your meal as well. If you have balanced foods and are still experiencing cravings, be sure you are drinking enough water. Dehydration can seem like hunger (remember Week 5? Of course you do!).

So, what do you crave and when do you crave it? An example of this might be—chocolate chip cookie dough ice cream at 10:30 p.m. while watching TV. I have *no idea* where I got the idea for that example . . .

Cravings I've experienced in the past seven days:

1. _____

_____

2. _____

_____

3. _____

_____

4. _____

_____

5. _____

_____

Now let's look at the reasons why you think you might be having these cravings. It is okay to self-diagnose your cravings based on our earlier detailed list. For example, that person who craved cookie dough ice cream might say: *I crave this at 10:30 p.m. because I skipped breakfast and my body is trying to make up for the missing calories.*

Or, other reasons could be

- I had a very salty and heavy dinner, so I crave something sweet and sugary at night.
- I skipped breakfast, lived on caffeine, and barely ate my lunch today.
- I didn't eat enough during the day, so my body is catching up late at night.
- I was so busy at work and forgot to bring my snacks with me, so I was starving when I got home.
- I had an argument with my significant other, so a glass or two of wine and something gooey and sweet seemed like a really good idea.
- I've only been getting five or six hours of sleep per night.
- I've been stress eating. I need to reduce my stress.
- I'm pretty sure I didn't drink any water today and only drank diet soda and coffee.
- I haven't been doing my regular exercise routine, so I feel terrible about myself and just want to eat junk food.
- I'm lonely and wish I had someone to cuddle up to rather than a pint of ice cream.

Why I think I am having my cravings:

1. _____

_____

2. _____

_____

3. _____

_____

4. _____

_____

5. _____

_____

Now that we've put on paper what you're craving and why you're craving it, let's come up with the solution. For example—At 10:30 p.m., I will remember to check my food log and commit to eating only the number of calories I have "left" in the day. So, I will substitute the cookie dough ice cream with a snack of almonds, berries, or five or six chocolate chips, which I will eat s-l-o-w-l-y (see our next section).

Other examples of how to conquer cravings

- I will get more sleep so I don't crave sweets, simple carbs, and caffeine.
- I will start eating breakfast.
- I will make sure I have snacks available at all times.
- I will make an effort to drink more water during the day rather than just coffee and diet sodas.
- I will make sure I eat something every three hours.
- When I feel the craving for sweets because of stress or loneliness, I will take a few deep breaths and make myself busy instead.
- I will get back to my regular exercise routine.
- I will allow myself a couple squares of dark chocolate after dinner to satisfy my sweet craving.
- I will start adding more "sweet" fruits and vegetables to my diet.
- I will cut down on my salt intake.
- I will make sure each meal has protein in it.
- I will eliminate all the junk food in my house so I'm not tempted anymore.
- I will drink water when I have a craving to see if it goes away, since I may just be dehydrated.

- I will make sure my meals have lots of color, which means I'll be getting more vitamins naturally in my diet.
- I will cut out all artificial sweeteners and switch to natural sweeteners instead.
- Instead of eating an entire bag of potato chips because I feel guilty for eating them in the first place, I will allow myself a single serving of chips to satisfy my craving.
- I will start bringing my lunch to work so I'm not tempted to eat out every day.

My solutions to get rid of my cravings:

1. _____
   _____

2. _____
   _____

3. _____
   _____

4. _____
   _____

5. _____
   _____

Good job! Once you realize the source of your cravings, it is very easy to reduce them.

MINDLESS EATING AND SPEED EATING

We've all done it—sat down in front of the computer or TV with food in our hands and, *poof*! It's gone! Do you even remember what you just ate? Do you remember how it tasted? We do this while driving also. We know there was a sandwich somewhere in the car, and now it has magically disappeared.

There is a subtle difference between *mindless eating*—eating without paying attention to what you are doing—and *speed eating*—eating too quickly—but they are closely related. So many of us eat without thinking *and* inhale our food within a couple of minutes.

The first technique to changing both mindless eating and speed eating is to slow down when you eat and actually look at your food. I don't mean stare at it or gaze at it lovingly, although you can certainly do that if you want. I mean really *see* what you are eating. What does it smell like? What does it look like? Delicious and tasty? Charred to a crisp? What sort of portion did you serve yourself? On a scale of 1 to 10 with 10 being the hungriest, how hungry are you?

The next trick is to try to not eat in front of the TV or the computer. You can DVR what you were watching on TV, and the computer will be waiting for you when you are done. Also, don't eat standing up. Sit down and actually enjoy your food. Put down your food in between bites. A sandwich or burger should touch the plate a few times while being eaten—not just hang in the air and dangle in your hand the whole time. Along the same lines, put down your utensils between bites. Don't just keep shoveling food into your mouth before you've barely swallowed the previous forkful.

When at home, it is important to sit and eat each meal at the table. If you eat with a significant other or your family, talk to each other and find out how the person's day was. Taking the time to talk to each other is important. There are so many distractions such as email, Facebook, cell phones, TV, computers ... sometimes people forget that the best form of communication is just talking to each other.

Okay, maybe I'm veering off topic as your health coach, but you know I'm right! I once went to dinner with my family to a fun hibachi restaurant where everyone was seated at one large table. I had never been to a hibachi restaurant before, so I was curious to see what it would be like to share a table with strangers. The family that sat next to us was a mom with two girls. One girl was about six years old and never looked up from her cell phone the entire meal. The other was about eight years old and put down her phone occasionally to put food in her mouth. Needless to say, they didn't talk much—to us or to each other.

Even if you live by yourself, turn off those distractions when you eat and just enjoy your meal. My mom recently commented to me that no matter what I'm doing or how busy I am, if I eat any meal, even just a snack, I eat sitting down. I never eat standing up or distracted, because I want to enjoy my food.

On the topic of mindless eating, sometimes I think people eat very quickly because there is an element of shame. We are embarrassed of what we are eating, so we eat it all as quickly as possible and act like it never happened. Let's pretend a person sits down for an ice cream sundae or just ordered a pizza. Instead of enjoying a few bites and calling it a day, the individual inhales the food as fast as possible because of guilt about eating it in the first place.

I know I have been guilty of binge eating in the past. When I was first trying to lose weight and was completely clueless about how to lose it correctly, I had some food issues. If I ate even one bite of a food I knew wasn't good for me—say, candy—I felt so guilty that I polished off the entire bag of candy in one sitting. Or box of cookies. Or container of sugar cereal. Or a whole pizza. Of course, this was when I didn't know anything about balance. I also didn't realize that the food wasn't going anywhere and that it didn't determine my worth. I now know that I am *worthy* of having a slice of pizza or a chocolate chip cookie here and there and saving some for tomorrow—it's not going anywhere.

Many people have food issues and not just the obvious ones like bingeing, anorexia, or bulimia. If you have kept your food log carefully, you know your body needs this food to live—so why not enjoy it? You will be amazed at how relaxing a meal can actually be when you are eating the right foods in the right amounts and paying attention to what you are eating. Conscious eating will transform your eating habits . . . and your body.

THE 20-MINUTE RULE

Did you know that it takes 20 minutes for the signal to go from your stomach to your brain to let you know you are full? That's right—20 whole minutes! Do you remember the last time it took you 20 minutes to eat your breakfast or lunch? I think most people eat breakfast in about 5 minutes. Most people probably eat dinner a bit slower, but everyone eats at a different pace. If you haven't heard about this scientific fact, now you know. There have been several studies that show overall caloric intake is decreased when a person eats more slowly.[10]

From the first moment food goes into your mouth, it takes about 20 minutes for it to be digested enough that glucose gets into the bloodstream and the hormones kick in. Hormones associated with digestion are insulin, leptin, cortisol, and ghrelin. They act as messengers between the stomach and the brain that give signals of satiety. You may eat all the food you need in 5 minutes, but your body still won't give you the "I'm stuffed" signal for another 15 minutes. That is why, if you are starving because you haven't eaten all day, and you inhale a large amount of food in just a few minutes, when the 20-minute mark comes around, you feel stuffed like a pig! You'll actually feel overstuffed because of the large amount of food you ate earlier. The reason for this is that you were technically "full" in those 5 minutes, but the "fullness signal" needed 15 more minutes to get to the brain, so you ate more than you needed to. Make sense?

This is another important reason to "see" your food so that you can learn the exact moment when you should stop eating. You can't figure

10 A. M. Andrade, G. W. Greene, and K. J. Melanson, "Eating Slowly Led to Decreases in Energy Intake within Meals in Healthy Women," *Journal of the Academy of Nutrition and Dietetics* 108, no. 7 (July 2008): 1186–91, doi:10.1016/j.jada.2008.04.026. PMID: 18589027.

out when this magical and life-altering moment happens if you are distracted. What you want to do is train yourself to stop eating the moment you feel slightly full.

When you sit down to start eating, you are generally very hungry, even starving—maybe around a 9 or 10 on a scale of 1 to 10. At some point, you will take a bite, swallow, and feel satiated. Not stuffed, but satiated. Your hunger level might then be at a 3 or 4. This is the magical moment when you should put down your fork and stop eating that meal. Let the stomach and brain communication catch up to the amount of food you have eaten.

BABY GOALS AND BABY STEPS

Unconscious eating puts on inches; conscious eating takes them off. In that spirit we turn to . . . yes, the three baby goals in reference to your cravings and the speed or mindlessness with which you eat.

Some sample baby goals for this week could be:

1. I won't eat in front of the TV anymore.
2. I'll eat at the dinner table, even if I eat by myself.
3. I won't eat standing up.

My three baby goals for this week are:

1. _____

   _____

2. _____

   _____

3. _____

   _____

We're coming into the home stretch! Two more weeks to go. Keep up the good work!

Week 8 Measurements

_____ Waist (1 in. above belly button)

_____ Hips (widest part around glutes)

_____ Lower abdomen (2 in. below BB)

_____ Right thigh (put right hand flat against leg and measure under the thumb area)

_____ Left thigh (put left hand flat against leg and measure under the thumb area)

_____ Chest (measure around widest part)

_____ Right arm (measure around bicep area)

_____ Left arm (measure around bicep area)

_____ Right calf (measure around widest part)

_____ Left calf (measure around widest part)

_____ INCHES LOST THIS WEEK

_____ CHANGE SINCE LAST WEEK

_____ TOTAL INCHES LOST SO FAR

WEEK 9

Like the Pros: Juicing, Going Organic, Vitamins and Supplements

How to *Not* Lose Your Mind: Lesson for Week 9

Whatever God put on the Earth is what you should eat. All those processed foods with impossible-to-pronounce ingredients that have eighteen letters per word should *not* go into our bodies. Pure and simple!

Now that you have made it to Week 9, you can definitely consider yourself "health conscious." You're exercising, you're paying attention to what you eat, and you're drinking enough water. You've probably lost some weight and more importantly, you've lost inches. Overall, I bet you are feeling much healthier. And yet . . . some of those darn fat cells still seem to be hanging around . . . literally.

TOXIC TOXINS

Fat cells are created a few different ways. One way, of course, is by eating more than you burn. Another way, which you may be completely unaware of, is by ingesting toxins. When the body absorbs toxins from the chemicals in foods and from the environment, those toxins are stored in our fat cells. There are fat-soluble toxins and water-soluble toxins. Fat-soluble toxins are heavy metals, parasites, pesticides, preservatives, food additives, pollutants, and other man-made toxins. Water-soluble toxins are flushed from the body through the blood and kidneys.

Why does the body store fat-soluble toxins in your fat cells? Because your body is trying to shield and protect you from the toxins; isn't that nice? How the body works is truly fascinating when you think about it. When the toxins become more concentrated in the body, the fat cells become larger in an effort to keep protecting you. The problem is, much of the time we don't think about it—instead we just give the body more and more toxins. Our bodies need a break!

How do we get rid of these toxins? Of the two main sources of toxins we just discussed, food and the environment, the first is much easier for us to control. You probably aren't planning to move out to the middle of nowhere where there is less pollution and the air is cleaner. What you can control easily is what you put into your body—what you eat and drink. I go by a simple rule of thumb—whatever God put on the Earth is what you should eat. When you ingest all those chemicals, the body has to work extra hard. When you eat what occurs naturally on this planet, it makes things easier on your body.

As a fun exercise, go grab one of your favorite snacks or "easy" dinners and look at the label. I'll wait. There are probably eighty-five ingredients listed and you have no idea what they are, let alone how to pronounce them! Just for kicks, make a list here of all of the ingredients you don't know how to pronounce:

Ingredients I can't pronounce but I'm pretty sure aren't natural foods:

1. _____

2. _____

3. _____

4. _____

5. _____

6. _____

7. _____

8. _____

9. _____

10. _____

For example, here are the ingredients in a candy bar. Just so you know, partially hydrogenated soybean and cottonseed oils are not natural, are unstable, and are *trans fats*, i.e., the fats that can clog arteries, lead to heart disease, and cause other problems.

Candy bar ingredients

Corn syrup, milk chocolate (milk chocolate contains: sugar, cocoa butter, chocolate, milk, lactose, milk fat, nonfat milk, and soya lecithin—an emulsifier), coconut, sugar, almonds, partially hydrogenated soybean and cottonseed oils, whey, salt, cocoa, vanilla, chocolate, soya lecithin and sodium metabisulfite to preserve color.

Let's try saying "sodium metabisulfite" three times, fast, shall we?

Now, here are the ingredients in a fast-food chain's hamburger. I don't know what all of these ingredients mean, but I sure don't want them in my body!

Fast-food hamburger ingredients

Beef, bun (flour enriched [Wheat Flour Bleached, Barley Malted Flour, Niacin, Iron Reduced, Thiamine Mononitrate (Vitamin B1), Ribofloavin (Vitamin B2), Folic Acid (Vitamin aB), Enzyme(s)], Water, Corn Syrup High Fructose, Sugar, Yeast, Soybean(s) Oil and/or, Soybean(s) Oil Partially Hydrogenated. Contains 2% or less of the Following: (Salt, Calcium Sulphate [Sulfate], Ammonium Sulfate, Calcium Carbonate, Calcium Propionate, Dough Conditioner(s) [Sodium Stearoyl Lactylate, Daten, Ascorbic Acid, Azodicarbonamide, mono and Diglycerides, Ethoxylated Monoglycerides, Monocalcium Phosphate, Enzyme(s), Guar Gum, Soy Flour, Calcium Peroxide], Sodium Propionate, Soy Lecithin, Wheat Gluten, Ammonium Chloride), Ketchup (Tomato(es) Concentrate, Vinegar Distilled, Corn Syrup High Fructose, Water, Corn Syrup, Salt, Flavor(s) Natural [Vegetable Sources]), Mustard (Vinegar Distilled, Water, Mustard Seed, Salt, Turmeric,

Paprika, Spice(s) Extractive), Pickle(s) (Cucumber(s), Water, Vinegar Distilled, Salt, Calcium Chloride, Alum, Potassium Sorbate Preservative, Flavor(s) Natural, Polysorbate 80, Turmeric Extratives, Onion(s) Chopped)

Now let's try saying "azodicarbonamide" three times, fast. By the way, azodicarbonamide is banned in the UK, most European countries, and Australia. I wonder why it is still legal in the US?

Here are the ingredients of an apple:
Apple

Here are the ingredients of water:
Water

Soooooo much simpler . . .

I realize that most of us probably can't eat unprocessed foods 100 percent of the time, but if we do our best, then that *will* be good enough. I go by the 90/10 rule; 90 percent of the time, I consume what I'm supposed to; 10 percent of the time, I do whatever I want.

DETOXING

Our bodies are naturally detoxing every day through sweat, through our kidneys, and through our liver. In simplest terms, it is important to sweat every day through exercise, to drink enough water until your urine is clear, and to have a bowel movement every day. You can see how all of these major bodily functions are important to help us detox. If you don't exercise, don't drink enough water, and are often constipated, you probably have a lot of toxins in your body that need to be eliminated. The more toxins you have, the harder it is for your body to lose inches, because it is not as efficient as it should be.

Even though these body systems are working as hard as they can, they often get overloaded and need a break. This is where a "cleanse" or a "detox" comes in—detox is short for "detoxification." Basically, it helps your body get rid of toxins in a concentrated and conscious way.

Here are some natural ways to help the body detox:

- Drink eight glasses (64 oz.) of water a day.
- Eliminate beverages like sodas (both regular and diet), alcohol, and caffeine.
- Add lemon or lime to your water.
- Have a teaspoon of apple cider vinegar a day (improves digestion and promotes alkalinity—get the kind of apple cider vinegar that contains the "mother").
- Eat lots of fiber (28 g per day for women and 35 g per day for men).
- Add more leafy greens.
- Drink herbal teas, such as decaf green tea.
- Quit smoking.

I would never jump into trying an official cleanse in the hopes of losing weight before cleaning up my diet and lifestyle first, nor would I recommend you do this, either. To naturally detox, I would first focus on eating a healthy diet, exercising, eating mostly unprocessed foods, and following the tips listed here. If you do want to try an official cleansing program, then I recommend consulting your doctor first. A person who has never done a cleanse before could experience many unpleasant side effects. If you currently drink alcohol and caffeine, eat a lot of fast food, don't exercise, smoke, etc., then going straight into a detox situation is not something I recommend. Side effects could include headaches, extreme fatigue, dizziness, irritability, nausea, vomiting, muscle pain, cramps, and even fever.

Therefore, it is best to clean up your diet *first* before trying a cleanse. Remember that the body is always naturally detoxing, so by just eating healthy and exercising, you will start to detox, lose weight, and lose inches without doing a formal "cleanse." Just eating a diet of mostly organic and unprocessed foods, as discussed in the next section, will benefit you further on your journey to losing inches.

After you've cleaned up your diet and consulted your doctor, there are a variety of different detoxes and cleanses available. Some of them are a bit rough on the system. I don't like anything with pills, as it has been my experience you'll spend a lot of time in the bathroom. I tried that water and maple syrup detox program and gave up quickly because I was *starving*. I've done colonics, which are interesting—not sure how I feel about those. I've also gone to a juicing retreat where I was starving and lightheaded for three days, lost water weight, and it all came back the second I ate real food. So, overall, I don't do formal cleanses anymore. All I do is make a super-duper juice concoction each morning, and then I make healthy choices throughout the day. Here is my favorite juicing recipe that I make almost every morning:

Justine's Favorite Juicing Recipe

1–2 apples

1–2 carrots

¼ wedge of lemon

½ cucumber

A handful of dark, leafy greens (kale, spinach, Swiss chard, or collards, etc.)

A bit of parsley

You can create any juicing combination you like. I probably make about 8 to 10 ounces of juice. The important thing is to get your *greens* in to start your day off right! I'll also put 1 or 2 teaspoons of omega-3 fish oil in there too. Sometimes I'll even add a scoop of "greens" powder in my juice. I drink my juice within a few minutes of making it, because the enzymes start to break down, and I want to make sure I get the full strength of the vitamins and nutrients. Dee-lish! Right after I drink my juice, I'll eat my breakfast.

By incorporating a juice drink in the morning, you'll set the tone for the day. Your kidneys, liver, and intestines will be happy, too. You'll also naturally make better food choices throughout the day, because your day began with such a healthy start.

ORGANIC FOODS VERSUS NATURAL FOODS

Over the past several years, there has been a tremendous movement toward purchasing and advocating organic products, natural products, and products that are better for the environment. With this inundation of information, however, comes a certain amount of confusion about what to actually purchase at the store. What does "organic" actually mean? Why do some food products have the USDA organic seal and others don't? Why do some products lack such a seal, but still read "organic"? And of course, the biggest question—which food products are really worth the extra money and which aren't?

As you read in the last section, when we have fewer toxins in our body, we have smaller fat cells, and to accomplish this we want to eat as little processed food as possible. Our bodies function best on a straight-from-the-earth diet. Now as it turns out, all-natural eating is good, but organic is better. Let's learn what natural versus organic means, as defined by the National Organic Program, which is a constituent of the USDA. Then you can make your own decisions about how to do your grocery shopping.

Natural Products

In general, the term *natural* can be used on products that are free of artificial ingredients such as chemicals or coloring preservatives. In addition, that food item and its ingredients must be only minimally processed. Natural foods may still carry some toxins due to being grown with synthetic pesticides and fertilizers, bioengineering, or irradiation.

Organic Products

Organic farming means that foods are grown without synthetic pesticides and fertilizers; although, organic farmers can still use natural pesticides and fertilizers. In 2002, the USDA enacted strict guidelines to
identify organic foods. Companies that produce foods that are organic
do not have to use the USDA organic label. However, companies that
use the label without certification can be fined up to $10,000.

To make matters a little more complicated, there are four different
levels to the organic designation:

- **100 percent Organic:** If you are going to go organic, 100
  percent is the way to go—but you knew I was going to say
  that! Products that say "100% Organic" must contain exactly
  that—100 percent organic ingredients. In addition, these products must have passed a government inspection. These products
  can use the USDA Organic seal on their label and in their
  advertisements.

- **Organic:** Products labeled as "organic" must contain at least
  95 percent organic ingredients. This is your second-best option
  when shopping for organic foods. These products must have
  passed a government inspection, and they are also allowed
  to use the USDA Organic seal on their products. The rest of
  the ingredients that are not organic must be on the nationally
  approved list put together by the National Organic Program.

- **70 percent Organic Ingredients:** Foods made with at least
  70 percent organic ingredients cannot put the USDA Organic
  Seal on their label. However, they can state "made with organic
  ingredients" on the label and list up to three such ingredients
  or food groups. The other 30 percent of ingredients must come
  from the nationally approved list of the National Organic Program. All products with 70 percent organic ingredients or more
  must also list the name and address of the government-approved
  certifying agent on the label.

- **Less than 70 percent Organic Ingredients:** Products using less than 70 percent organic ingredients cannot use the USDA seal, nor can they make any organic claims on their label. They are only allowed to list any organic ingredients on the side of the label.

Now that you know the difference between natural and organic foods and the different levels of "organic" available, it makes it easier when it comes to decisions at the grocery store. However, a question may arise: What if it is too expensive to go 100 percent organic all at once? Where should I start?

The first place I would start is by shopping the outer perimeter of the grocery store. This is where your healthiest foods are. Try to purchase only organic fruits and vegetables. Yes, it may be a few dollars more, but you'll be healthier for it and will find the savings by limiting future health problems and doctor visits. Plus, your food will taste so much better that it will be easier to stick to a lower calorie, higher nutrient diet.

If you can't afford all organic fruits and vegetables, then you can opt to buy conventionally (non-organically) those fruits and veggies that have a thick outer skin—e.g., oranges, grapefruits, bananas, avocados, etc. The outer layer adds a little more protection from herbicides and pesticides compared to lettuce, for example, which has no protection. Ideally, however, you want to buy all organic produce.

Have you ever noticed how a strawberry just doesn't taste the same any more? If you try a regular, conventionally grown strawberry, they have no taste. Then if you try an organic or locally grown strawberry, they are sweet and delicious, just like they should be! Conventional produce is grown using so many pesticides and herbicides that you may unintentionally be harming your health. Other conventional produce may also be genetically modified (GMO) or altered—there are over fifty such GMO products approved in the United States. Consider staying away from products with GMO on their labels.

There are many unknowns as to the long-term health effects of consuming such items.

Other products I think are essential to buy organic are meat, eggs, milk, and poultry. When buying these products, look for the words "raised without added hormones" or "raised without added antibiotics." These statements are allowed by the Food Safety and Inspection Service of the USDA. Companies are not allowed to put the words "hormone free" or "antibiotic free" on their labels. Why? I don't know, but those are the rules. Why is it important to buy products without added hormones or antibiotics? Ever wonder why girls are starting to develop breasts so early, and why some get their periods as young as seven or eight years old? It is in part due to the added hormones in their foods and milk. These added hormones just aren't necessary. Why put additional hormones in our bodies and in our kids' bodies that aren't natural?

When buying fish, it is important to buy *wild* fish. These fish generally have less mercury in them. Refer to pages 82 to 83 for a complete list of which fish have the least and most mercury. The best types of wild salmon are wild Alaskan or sockeye salmon. It has the least amount of mercury (second to scallops) and is very high in omega-3s. What's wrong with mercury? As we previously learned, it is a heavy metal that can attach to the major organs and slowly cause them to shut down. Pregnant women should avoid fish that are high in mercury, because it has been linked to autism.

To get the greatest variety of organic options, I recommend adding a health food store or a health-conscious chain grocery store to your weekly food-shopping itinerary. Many regular grocery stores now contain an organic section, which is awesome. They may not have the variety that a bigger health food store does, but it's a start!

Your best bet for saving some bucks on delicious, organic foods is visiting a farmer's market. You'll be supporting local farmers and picking up the best in-season foods your area has to offer. Better yet, the person you buy your goods from will be able to tell you how the food was grown and harvested in addition to giving you tips on different ways to prepare it. Trust me, there's nothing like a tomato that's just been pulled off the vine!

Depending on where you live, you may also be able to join a co-op. Once you become a member (some charge a monthly fee while others charge per delivery) you'll receive several pounds of the seasonal fruits, vegetables, and other farm-grown goods that are currently being harvested. Want to find a farmer's market or co-op near you? Go to www.localharvest.org and www.coopdirectory.org to find out more.

Every time you are in the checkout line at a grocery store or go to a farmer's market, you are casting your vote. Remember that buying organic is a vote for your health, for the environment, and for local farmers. Why do you think so many grocery stores and large-chain stores now offer organic options? Because of *you*. Every purchase that you make is a vote, and your votes have been heard!

VITAMINS AND SUPPLEMENTS

Many people frequently ask me if I think it is a good idea to take vitamins and supplements. Well . . . I think it *could* be a good idea if a person is not eating a balanced enough diet. The easiest thing—and the cheapest thing—is to eat a variety of fresh, organic foods that are not processed and therefore have little to no toxins, so that you get all your vitamins and minerals naturally.

Your refrigerator can be your "medicine cabinet." Dark, leafy greens contain many vitamins and minerals such as vitamin K, vitamin C, calcium, and iron; mushrooms are high in magnesium and zinc; carrots have vitamin A; bananas have potassium . . . the list goes on and on. You can look at the USDA's National Agricultural Library (http://ndb.nal.usda.gov) to do a search and see which vitamins and minerals are contained in your favorite foods.

I take very few supplements and am rarely sick, so I must be getting the proper nutrients in my diet. The only supplements I take are a whole-food multivitamin, omega-3s, and a liquid B12 complex. In the winter months, I'll also take vitamin D. The multivitamin I like is a whole-food multivitamin, which can be purchased at a health food store or in the health section of your grocery store. Seeing the words "whole food" on the label means it is actually made from food! Cheaper multivitamins may lack the same quality ingredients, so your body may not digest and absorb them as well. In fact, they may go right through you, which is just putting your money down the toilet . . . literally. So, when reading the label of your next multivitamin, make sure it says "whole food."

We talked about omega-3s and how important they are to incorporate into your daily regimen in Week 6. Again, they come in liquid or gelcap form. See page 81 for more details about omega-3s.

For vitamin D, I prefer either sublingual (it dissolves under the tongue) or liquid. These two forms are more efficient and get into the bloodstream faster. Vitamin D is essential for bone health, a healthy immune system, regulating blood pressure, helping prevent autoimmune disorders, and aiding absorption of calcium and phosphorous. If you get sick often, are tired all the time, are depressed, or are trying to prevent osteoporosis, take vitamin D! The best thing, however, is to get out in the sunlight. Go outside in the sun each day for 5 to 15 minutes without sunblock, particularly between 10:00 a.m. and 3:00 p.m. during the spring, summer, and fall. During the winter, longer exposure may be needed, because the sun's rays are weaker.

As I mentioned, I take a B12 complex in liquid form every day—just a few dropperfuls under the tongue. If you have stress in your life, B vitamins are nature's de-stressors! When you feel stressed, you actually urinate out your B vitamins, because they are water soluble. B12 is the only B vitamin that is fat soluble and can be stored in the body. In addition to reducing stress, B12 is important for DNA synthesis, red blood cell production, a healthy nervous system, and fat and protein metabolism. It also gives you a natural energy boost. Coffee? No way. I take my B vitamins.

The best thing to do if you are considering taking additional supplements is to first consult a doctor, a nutritionist, or a registered dietician. There are so many vitamins and supplements out there that it can be really confusing. It is also possible to over-supplement and actually poison the body. It is better to be safe than sorry and educate yourself on what you are about to put into your body. Learn what the supplement can do for you, how it can possibly harm you if you take too much, and what the best dosage is for you based on your health history and age. So, before you decide to supplement, ask your doctor or a nutrition professional.

BABY GOALS AND BABY STEPS

Phew! We sure did cover a lot this week. You might have gathered some ideas for actions you want to take in the future, but I would never advocate you try everything all at once. However, it is important to put something into action, so how about it? What are your baby steps for this week? Are you going to venture for the first time into the organic section of the supermarket? Or, are you going to dig out your juicer and clean out the cobwebs?

Some sample baby goals for this week could be:

1. I will clean out the pantry and refrigerator of foods that have chemical-laden ingredients I can't pronounce.
2. I will shop for organic foods more often.
3. I will try Justine's favorite juicing recipe in the morning.

My three baby goals for this week are:

1. _____

   _____

2. _____

   _____

3. _____

   _____

Only one more week... almost there! I can taste the celebratory organic juice concoction from here—which, of course, you are drinking while wearing your skinny jeans!

Week 9 Measurements

_____Waist (1 in. above belly button)

_____Hips (widest part around glutes)

_____Lower abdomen (2 in. below BB)

_____Right thigh (put right hand flat against leg and measure under the thumb area)

_____Left thigh (put left hand flat against leg and measure under the thumb area)

_____Chest (measure around widest part)

_____Right arm (measure around bicep area)

_____Left arm (measure around bicep area)

_____Right calf (measure around widest part)

_____Left calf (measure around widest part)

_____INCHES LOST THIS WEEK

_____CHANGE SINCE LAST WEEK

_____TOTAL INCHES LOST SO FAR

WEEK 10

Maintain the Magic

How to *Not* Lose Your Mind: Lesson for Week 10

Yes, it *is* possible to lose your inches *and* keep them off during the holidays, while traveling, when going on vacation, and while enjoying all that life has to offer. Maintaining the magic is possible—the key is to find your *balance*.

Have you ever started a diet or an exercise program and quit after a period of a few days or a few weeks? Okay, that question is kind of a joke—we all have, innumerable times! The real question is, do you know *why* you fell off the exercise or diet bandwagon? Chances are excellent that it was because one of your Primary Foods was out of balance.

PRIMARY FOODS

The term "Primary Food"[11] may not be one you are familiar with. It's a concept I learned about when I attended the Institute for Integrative Nutrition°. Primary Foods are not actual foods—they are instead other factors that affect our overall health. The idea is that there are certain influences aside from what you put on your plate or how often you move your body that affect your health.

Primary Foods are (1) physical activity, (2) career, (3) relationships, and (4) spirituality. When one or more of our Primary Foods are off-kilter, it can create a void that we often try to fill with food and

---

self-defeating activities. No amount of chocolate cake or sinking farther into the couch will fix a troubled relationship or an unfulfilling career.

Let's explore how these four Primary Food groups can affect our bodies.

Physical Activity

We've certainly talked about this quite a bit in the book. It all comes down to exercise. Our bodies are made to move, and our muscles are made to be used. Not getting enough exercise? Maybe it's because you haven't found something you enjoy. Enjoying the activity is the key. This leads to more movement and more happiness, which creates more balance in our lives. If you haven't figured out what you love yet, then keep trying new things until you do!

Not exercising because you're feeling pressed for time? Just start with 10 minutes of activity a day. Soon enough, you'll be exercising more and more and it will become second nature.

Career

Here's one simple question: Do you like your job? Do you like what you do each day? If the answer is no, then it's time to see what you can do about it. Are you in a position to quit and pursue what you love? Or do you need to stay where you are—for now—while you start looking for a new job? Can you take some night classes to pursue another career? Do you like most of your responsibilities, but think you could improve upon a few areas? Do you like your coworkers and your office environment?

When you are happy in your career, it honestly just makes your life easier, happier, and healthier. A wise man (i.e., my dad) once told me, "Do what you love because then you'll never work a day in your life!" That is exactly how I feel about what I do now. However, I have to say I've had plenty of jobs where I literally felt like I was in the movie *Office Space*. If you haven't seen the movie, it's really funny. It's about feeling like you're in prison each day at work; you just stare at the clock, counting down the minutes until you can leave.

When you are unhappy with your day job, it makes you feel irritable and grumpy, and you take out your misery on your loved ones. You may also not sleep well, and you don't really look forward to each day, because you know what to expect. In my first job out of college, I remember I cried a few times the night before going to work because I hated my job so much. Eventually I was able to quit and found something new, but boy, I was sure miserable at the time! Unhappiness like this leads to worse food choices because, hey, who cares? It can also lead to mindless eating at work to give you something to do or to take your mind off your humdrum day job. Waking up each morning and knowing you get to do what you love will change your life and your health—for the better!

Relationships

From parents to siblings to best friends, acquaintances, and significant others, our lives are filled with different kinds of relationships. When we're feeling unfulfilled in our relationships, it is easy to turn to food (or drink) in times of stress. Is that healthy? Definitely not!

It's time to think about your relationships productively. Consider which ones you are happy with and which ones make you feel incomplete, unworthy, or stressed. Is there any way to improve that relationship? Or would it be best to let it go?

We can't change others; we can only change ourselves. Never feel that you can "fix" a relationship by trying to change another person. From my own personal experience, I know that it won't happen, and you'll completely exhaust yourself. Making the choice to end an unfulfilling relationship may be difficult, but it's worth it.

Spirituality

Spirituality in general is different for every person. It could be anything from going to church, to meditating, to spending time in nature, to doing yoga, or to reading an enlightening book. If you feel that you would be happier and healthier with more spirituality in your life, brainstorm how to increase your intake of this Primary Food group in ways that are appealing to you.

Now, take a moment to address each Primary Food in your life, whether it needs a little improvement or a lot. For example, when evaluating the Primary Food group "career," your entry might look like this:

> I hate my job and am miserable every day.

Then brainstorm your next steps, such as:

1. Redo resume.
2. Apply for five positions online each week.
3. Use word-of-mouth to try to secure a new job.
4. Go back to school/take night classes.

An example of your entry for "relationships" might read something like this:

> Overall I feel pretty solid in my connections with my loved ones, but I want to do even more with them.

Then your next steps to take might be:

1. Spend more time with my children.
2. Spend at least 10 minutes a day with my significant other to catch up.
3. Share the healthy food I am now cooking with a friend or family member and drop off a surprise delivery.

Or, on a different note, your example for "relationships" may even look like this:

> I'm miserable in my relationship and don't know how to fix it or end it.

Then your steps might look like this:

1. Talk to my partner about my concerns and see what s/he says.
2. Work on better communication.
3. Decide if I want to stay in this relationship.
4. Take action—leave or stay.

Take a moment to examine the four Primary Food groups next. Write down how you feel about each area and the steps you can take to improve them.

Primary Food 1: Physical Activity

How I feel about where I am now: _____

_____

_____

_____

Steps to take to improve this area:

1. _____

_____

2. _____

_____

3. _____

_____

Primary Food 2: Career

How I feel about where I am now: _____

_____

_____

_____

Steps to take to improve this area:

1. _____

_____

2. _____

_____

3. _____

_____

Primary Food 3: Relationships

How I feel about where I am now: _____

_____

_____

_____

Steps to take to improve this area:

1. _____

_____

2. _____

_____

3. _____

_____

Primary Food 4: Spirituality

How I feel about where I am now: _____

_____

_____

_____

Steps to take to improve this area:

1. _____

_____

2. _____

_____

3. _____

_____

MAINTAINING THE MAGIC

Once you have addressed the needs of your Primary Food groups, you will find that it is much easier to exercise, eat thoughtfully, and plan your days with a focus on your overall health . . . you may even find that you have the tools in place to maintain the magic forever!

Now that you've taken action to embrace a healthy lifestyle, apparent "trouble spots" such as eating out, parties, vacations, and holidays can be addressed with the same principles we have learned throughout this program, so that you are able to conquer both large and small obstacles.

A Typical Day

I've worked 9-to-5 jobs and flexible jobs, so I know that no matter what your work schedule is, the key to maintaining the magic during the workweek is *planning*.

Right now, my schedule varies from day to day, but no matter what time I wake up, the routine doesn't change. After I wake up, I feed my dog and cats, wash up, and then automatically head to the kitchen— even if I'm still half asleep—because I know breakfast is the most important meal of the day. We've already covered this, right? Right!

Your metabolism doesn't wake up until you eat something, so if you want to burn more calories during the day, you must eat something early. You have to have something in your stomach every single morning—period. I always eat breakfast within 15 to 20 minutes of hopping out of bed, but make sure you eat within that 45-minute window.

I find it useful to have three different options for what I will eat for breakfast in the back of my mind:

- The **Running Late Option**—This option happens more often than not! In this situation, I will either make a little gluten-free toast with organic peanut or almond butter and raw honey and eat it in the car, grab a protein bar, make a quick protein shake or smoothie, grab some hard-boiled eggs, or pack up my cereal or oatmeal so I can make it at work and eat a banana in the car.

- The **Wake-Up-In-Time Option**—I'm still half asleep, but I'm not feeling rushed for time. When this is the case, I eat some high-fiber or gluten-free cereal with unsweetened almond or cashew milk. I drizzle a little raw honey on my cereal for some sweetness and occasionally throw in some blueberries, raspberries, or chia seeds. When I'm in the mood for something hot, oatmeal is my go-to option. I choose plain, steel-cut oats or Irish oatmeal, swirl in a tablespoon of organic peanut butter to make it gooey and creamy, and add a little cinnamon.

- The **I'm-Having-a-Very-Relaxing-Morning Option**—For those rare times when I have some time to enjoy being home, I'll cook up two free-range eggs over easy and have a slice of gluten-free toast with a small pat of real butter.

See pages 40 to 41 for more quick and healthy breakfast options.

Now you've left the house . . . which is where all your food is! This is where *planning* gets really important. Before I grab my purse and hit the road, I have to think about my snacks and meals for the rest of the day. Do I need to bring a lunch? What snacks are sitting in my desk drawer? Do I have my water bottle? When I'm rushing out the door, I quickly consider where I'll be during the day and how I want to eat. I always have food on me! My family actually gets the biggest kick from this. If we are somewhere and somebody gets hungry, they know to ask me for munchies. Before I walk out the door, I'll grab snacks like an apple, pear, berries, grapes, a protein bar, a handful of nuts, or I'll even make a quick turkey sandwich to eat later.

If I know I'll be somewhere that may not have good lunch choices, I'll quickly put together something for lunch. Typically it is something ready-made that I have in the fridge, like leftovers, some sort of meat or fish that I'll put on salad, homemade egg salad with rice crackers, homemade chili or soup, or a low sodium turkey, mustard, and lettuce wrap on a gluten-free tortilla. I always bring a little more food than I may need during the day, just in case I'm in a location lacking healthy options.

I try to keep dinner simple. Sometimes it's leftovers with salad or fresh vegetables. Other times it's a portion of protein and some green vegetables. On occasion, it could even be an omelet with whatever veggies I have in the refrigerator. When I want to wind down at the end of the day, simple meals always win. I'm a functional and practical eater—when I'm hungry, I want something quick and healthy.

Dessert is the meal I look forward to the most. I indulge my sweet tooth with one square of dark chocolate or a small handful of super-dark chocolate chips every day. Sometimes I will have strawberries, blueberries, or raspberries for dessert.

If you have a family or a significant other who also wants to be healthy, you'll have to plan a little more than an individual would. If you have kids, make sure there are healthy snacks available for after school. Have cut-up fresh vegetables ready to go in the fridge with some hummus, sliced turkey, peanut butter and celery, apples, pears, sliced melon, grapes . . . think quick and healthy when it comes to snacks. The same thing also goes for adults—always have healthy snacks available in the fridge for when you come home after work and are hungry. What you see when you first open the refrigerator is what you will eat. Put the healthy foods up front and hide the not-so-healthy foods in the back.

Both adults and children will be healthier by bringing their lunch to work or school. That way you can control what you and your children are eating—plus you will save money. For healthy dinner options, plan ahead. Each morning, I always think about what I want for dinner so that if I need to thaw out some protein such as chicken or fish, it will be ready to cook when I come home. Add a salad or some steamed veggies, and you have a perfectly healthy dinner!

Think About It

Take a moment and figure out exactly what foods you need to bring with you before you walk out the door in the morning.

Breakfast options: _____

_____

_____

_____

Mid-morning snack options: _____

_____

_____

_____

Lunch options: _____

_____

_____

_____

Afternoon snack options: _____

_____

_____

_____

Dinner options: _____

_____

_____

_____

TIME FOR FUN!

When fun things come up in your life, it's important to be able to enjoy them. Getting hung up on eating perfectly or sticking to your healthy food plan can put a damper on an evening out. Living the good life is all about finding your *balance*.

I said *balance*, folks! Some people think special events like parties, dates, or a night out are a free pass to eat and drink whatever they want. Not true.

The most important thing is to give your exercise plan a boost on the day of a social event. Make a commitment to do your regular exercise routine plus a little extra. Then, when you're at the party munching on finger foods, you'll be happy knowing that you burned some extra calories earlier in the day—you may even choose more wisely having been inspired by your previous actions.

Regarding Alcohol . . .

We already covered this in Week 5. Overall, watch the alcohol. If your inches are not shrinking as quickly as you'd like, re-examine your alcohol intake.

Think About It

If you are planning a fun night out and intend to enjoy a few cocktails, it is helpful to learn (and remember!) how many calories are in each drink. We all have our favorites, so it's time for you to do a quick calculation and look at the labels to see how many calories are in each drink.

My Favorite Drinks:	Calories per Drink:
1.	
2.	
3.	
4.	
5.	

Going Out to Eat

One of life's pleasures is going out for a nice meal with friends and family. There's no reason you can't enjoy yourself while losing your inches, as long as you consume everything in moderation. Eating out multiple times a week can make it difficult to rein in temptation, so I try to make dining out a treat instead of a commonplace activity.

In the past few years, there have been major changes on restaurant menus to make dining out healthfully much easier. By law, restaurants with more than twenty locations are required to post the nutrition information for every meal they offer. Finding out what your favorite dish contains can be a real eye-opener—and not necessarily in a good way! I have seen salads with 1,500 calories and over 1,000 mg of sodium. So, even though it's a salad, it may not be the best option—you have to look at the nutrition information. Requiring restaurants to post nutritional information has caused them to be more diligent about their ingredients in order to attract diners. This helps us as consumers to plan meals that will help us meet our goals.

If you know in advance where you are going to eat, visit the restaurant's website and take a peek at the menu. If you can't do that, you can still make wise choices when you order. Substituting fresh veggies for french fries, asking for salad dressing on the side, and choosing grilled meats over breaded ones can cut out a lot of calories and fat.

Some other healthy habits you can try when dining out are to ignore the bread basket, share an appetizer or salad, and/or even split an entree. Eat only until you are satiated (a level 3 or 4 on the hunger scale) and then take home leftovers. When it's time for dessert, order one for the table so everyone can have a few fulfilling bites.

Remember, being picky is a good thing. Tell the server *exactly* what you want. After all, you are the one purchasing the meal, so you might as well eat exactly what you want and how you want it!

Here is a list of words that you *want* to look for in your food selection as well those you *don't want*:

Want		Don't Want	
Baked	Vegetarian	Fried	Battered
Grilled	Vinaigrette	Breaded	Crunchy
Steamed	High-fiber	Buttered	White sauce
Fresh	Whole-grain	Cheesy	Casserole
Roasted	Marinated	Loaded	Hollandaise
Boiled	Multi-grain	Smothered	Au gratin
Broiled	Seasoned	Stuffed	Country-style
Light	Poached (if not poached in duck fat)	Creamy	Basted
		Crispy	Stroganoff

Vacation

I'm happiest when I'm traveling, so making a vacation work with my health plan is a must. The best thing to do is to get into a healthy routine *now* so that when vacation comes around, you don't have to do anything different. Just keep doing what you're doing and your waistline will stay the same. Nonetheless, vacations can be challenging, so to meet this challenge, I like to break down an upcoming trip into three parts: before, during, and after.

Before Vacation

People are usually gung-ho about weight loss before vacation, because they've already decided that they'll "let it all go" during the vacation itself. But . . . why? Why is it that when we are on vacation, we decide to eat absolutely everything, drink every day, and sit around and do nothing? A vacation can be healthy without sacrificing a second of fun.

Here's a secret: Cutting down before you take a trip will help you stick to your food plan while on vacation. Start at least a month or earlier before you hit the road, especially if you're heading to a swimsuit-mandatory locale. Limiting your drinking helps you trim your waistline while decreasing your tolerance, which will help you drink less for the same feeling when you're on vacation. Planning meals and controlling portion sizes will help you begin to realize how much food you should be eating and will help you to stop eating once you've reached your limit.

Set a goal to exercise *at least* three times a week before going on vacation. Aim for at least 30 minutes of cardio and two to three days of resistance training.

During Vacation

I think the best thing to do during vacation is to get in a little activity right after you wake up. That way, you can enjoy the rest of the day doing whatever you want and you won't feel bad if you never move from your pool chair. Do everyone else a favor and get them to move, too! There are tons of easy ways to get yourself out and about. Walk on the beach, take advantage of your hotel's fitness center, or explore the town you're staying in.

After Vacation

When you return home, resist the urge to step on the scale. If you've been conscientious about exercising and eating well, you won't see a change in your size. You may see an increase on the scale due to water weight or actual weight if you overindulged, so give yourself a week or two before you step on the scale. If you've been a little lax, pinning a number to it will only make you feel worse. Resume your everyday healthy eating and exercise schedule and you'll be back to normal in no time.

Think About It

Take a moment to write down what you typically do before, during, and after vacation. Then write down a few things you may want to do differently next time.

What I usually do:

Before: _____

_____

_____

During: _____

_____

_____

After: _____

_____

_____

What I'm going to do now:

Before: _____

_____

_____

During: _____

_____

_____

After: _____

_____

_____

Holidays

The holidays can be tough because of all the temptation. First, there is the food. With the onslaught of traditional holiday foods, gifts of food, and those sugar cookies your kids just decorated, it's so easy to over-indulge. Allow yourself a few bites of your favorite holiday food, and then stick to a healthier eating plan. If you can't fight the temptation of edible gifts—i.e., if you find yourself eating pie for breakfast—do yourself a favor and stop! Send guests home with goodies or get rid of the leftover pie that is tempting you. Consider your weaknesses when it comes to your favorite holiday foods. Decide which indulgences are worth it and which you can leave off your dinner plate.

As always, the most important tool you can use to battle overindul-gence with food, besides your willpower, is to remain consistent with exercise. Working out just three times a week, even when the holidays make your daily schedule more hectic than usual, can make all the difference. You will naturally make better choices all around ... and those inches will continue to melt off your waistline—or at least you will maintain your pre-holiday size.

Besides food, the second biggest problem that people face every year during the holidays is *stress*. Shopping for gifts, decorations, and last-minute groceries can be extremely stressful. You now know that stress can cause you to crave sweets, junk food, and fast food. We've talked about how it can also increase your blood pressure and cause belly-fat producing cortisol to build up in your body. Here are a few more of my best stress-relief tips to help you stay calm this holiday season:

- **Always have snacks with you.** Chances are you will be shopping a lot longer than intended, and suddenly the food court in the mall will seem like a great idea. Besides, if your blood sugar is dropping, you are probably not making very good choices about what you are eating.

- **Pick a day and time when the stores will be the least crowded.** If necessary, take a half-day off from work if you can. I have found that shopping in the morning or early afternoon on weekdays is the most productive.

- **Expect chaos, and don't let it faze you.** When it happens, as it always does, you'll be focused on selecting the perfect present instead of chewing out the guy who cut you off.

- **Be friendly to sales associates.** I always make a point to try and make the person smile if he or she seems extra-stressed. You'll get better service and improve someone else's day.

- **Listen to classical or holiday music in your car.** Ever wonder why busy airports and train and subway stations play relaxing music? Because it *works*. NYC's Penn Station, one of the busiest stations in the United States, plays classical music. I should know, because I would listen to it daily when I worked in NYC. It was surprisingly relaxing.

- **Remember the spirit of the season.** It's not about how much you get or give to someone—it's the thought that counts! The best thing about the holidays is spending time with your family and the people you care about. The greatest gift you can give someone is your time.

Think About It

It's time to revise your own holiday routine. Use the lines here to outline the typical problems you face during the holidays. Include those foods you can limit or omit from your diet.

My typical issues during the holiday season:

1. _____

   _____

2. _____

   _____

3. _____

   _____

What I'm going to do about it this holiday season:

1. _____

   _____

2. _____

   _____

3. _____

   _____

THE FINISH LINE! CONGRATULATIONS!

You made it! How do you feel? Aren't you *proud* of yourself? You should be. Most people can't commit to anything for ten days, let alone ten weeks. I know that by now you have lost inches, you are looking better, and you are feeling good about yourself—all without losing your mind! Don't you feel sane and grateful to know that living a healthy lifestyle doesn't have to be so complicated? It's simple once you break it down into baby steps. You are now living a healthier lifestyle, which is the biggest accomplishment of all!

Let's take a final measurement, shall we? Be sure to compare Week 1 with Week 10 and be proud of the progress you have made.

Week 10 Measurements

_____ Waist (1 in. above belly button)

_____ Hips (widest part around glutes)

_____ Lower abdomen (2 in. below BB)

_____ Right thigh (put right hand flat against leg and measure under the thumb area)

_____ Left thigh (put left hand flat against leg and measure under the thumb area)

_____ Chest (measure around widest part)

_____ Right arm (measure around bicep area)

_____ Left arm (measure around bicep area)

_____ Right calf (measure around widest part)

_____ Left calf (measure around widest part)

_____ INCHES LOST THIS WEEK

_____ CHANGE SINCE LAST WEEK

TOTAL INCHES LOST OVERALL
_____ (WEEK 1 to WEEK 10)

CONCLUSION

Now that you have lost inches and are feeling healthier, I hope you are feeling more confident, mentally and physically, about how you can *Lose Your Inches without Losing Your Mind* and keep them off. I have given you *all* my secrets. I feel as though we've become good friends throughout this whole process!

You have learned, in no particular order:

How to break up with your scale.

How to count and keep a food log.

That baby goals and baby steps are your best friends.

How much you should eat during the day and how often.

Why eating every three hours will change your life and your waistline.

Why eating breakfast is really, really, really important, and when to eat it.

Why artificial sweeteners are terrible for you.

Why protein, carbs, and fats are important, and the differences between them.

How to naturally rid your body of toxins.

Why it is important to drink water.

How to incorporate exercise into your life, why it is important, and how to make it fun and stick to it.

What organic means and why it's important.

Which vitamins and supplements may be beneficial.

Why juicing in the morning is a good idea.

How to figure out why you are craving something and what your body is telling you.

How to eat slower and enjoy your food rather than devour it in a few seconds.

Why it is important to be happy in all aspects of your life, including Primary Foods—physical activity, career, relationships, and spirituality.

How to maintain the magic while dining out, going to parties and social events, while on vacation, and during the holidays.

My hope for you is that you keep this book handy in your purse, bag, or briefcase, and take things one step at a time. Reread each chapter if you need to, and be sure to do all the steps. I *know* you can keep losing those inches and I *know* that you now have all the tools to make it happen! The rest is up to you. If I can do it, so can you.

I am your number-one supporter. I look forward to hearing your success stories and *I'm proud of you already* for taking these steps to *Lose Your Inches without Losing Your Mind!*

Your Friend in Health (and Mental Happiness),

Justine

APPENDIX I

Nutrition Chart

Here is a quick reference chart of popular healthy food items in each major category.

FISH

Food	Amount	Calories	Protein (g)	Fat (g)	Carbs (g)	Fiber (g)	Sodium (mg)
Anchovies, in olive oil, drained	3 pieces	12	2	0	0	0	200
Atlantic croaker	3 ounces	88	15	3	0	0	48
Atlantic haddock	3 ounces	95	21	1	0	0	74
Bass (striped)	3 ounces	105	19	3	0	0	75
Butterfish	3 ounces	159	19	9	0	0	97
Catfish	3 ounces	89	16	2	0	0	42
Cod	3 ounces	89	19	1	0	0	66
Crab, Alaskan king	3 ounces	82	16	1	0	0	911
Crab, Dungeness	3 ounces	93	19	1	1	0	321
Crawfish	3 ounces	70	14	1	0	0	80
Flounder	3 ounces	99	21	1	0	0	89
Hake	3 ounces	61	13	0	0	0	72
Halibut	3 ounces	119	23	2	0	0	59
Herring	3 ounces	173	20	10	0	0	98
Lobster (spiny)	3 ounces	122	22	2	3	0	193
Mackerel	3 ounces	223	20	15	64	0	71
Mahi Mahi	3 ounces	93	16	0	0	0	96

Fish, continued

Food	Amount	Calories	Protein (g)	Fat (g)	Carbs (g)	Fiber (g)	Sodium (mg)
Mullet	3 ounces	128	21	4	0	0	60
Oysters	3 ounces	50	5	1	5	0	151
Perch (ocean)	3 ounces	103	20	2	0	0	82
Pollock	3 ounces	100	21	1	0	0	94
Salmon	3 ounces	184	23	9	0	0	56
Sardines, in water	1 can	140	19	7	0	0	270
Scallops (steamed)	3 ounces	93	18	0	0	0	222
Salmon (canned), no salt	3 ounces	116	19	4	0	0	64
Sea bass (Chilean)	3 ounces	105	20	2	0	0	74
Sole	3 ounces	99	21	1	0	0	89
Squid, calamari, raw	3 ounces	78	13	1	2	0	37
Tilapia	3 ounces	109	22	2	0	0	48
Trout (freshwater)	3 ounces	128	19	5	0	0	48
Tuna (skipjack)	3 ounces	112	24	1	0	0	40
Tuna, canned light chunk in water	3 ounces	99	22	1	0	0	287
Whiting	3 ounces	99	20	1	0	0	112

POULTRY

Food	Amount	Calories	Protein (g)	Fat (g)	Carbs (g)	Fiber (g)	Sodium (mg)
Chicken breast (skinless)	3 ounces	138	27	3	0	0	63
Chicken, dark meat, no skin	3 ounces	150	21	6	0	0	81
Chicken, oven roasted, deli	1 ounce	25	5	0	0	0	170
Duck, roasted, without skin	3 ounces	171	20	9	0	0	55
Turkey, light meat, no skin	3 ounces	119	25	1	0	0	48
Turkey burger patty	1 patty	180	21	9	0	0	100
Turkey, oven roasted, deli	1 slice	22	3	0	0	0	213
Turkey, dark meat, no skin	3 ounces	138	24	3	0	0	67

BEEF/PORK/LAMB

Food	Amount	Calories	Protein (g)	Fat (g)	Carbs (g)	Fiber (g)	Sodium (mg)
Bacon, reduced sodium	1 piece	43	3	3	0	0	82
Bison, ground	3 ounces	142	17	8	0	0	45
Bison, steak	3 ounces	180	21	11	0	0	41
Beef, ground, 95% lean	3 ounces cooked	164	25	6	0	0	72
Beef, hamburger patty	¼ lb burger	290	19	23	0	0	75
Beef ribs, small, trimmed to 0% fat	3 ounces	212	23	13	0	0	48
Ham, deli, extra lean	1 slice	29	5	1	0	0	286
Lamb, chop	1 small	112	14	5	0	0	210

Beef/Pork/Lamb, continued

Food	Amount	Calories	Protein (g)	Fat (g)	Carbs (g)	Fiber (g)	Sodium (mg)
Lamb, leg	3 ounces	153	24	5	0	0	56
Meatball, beef	1 small	40	2	2	0	0	38
Meatball, turkey	1 small	49	5	2	2	0	162
Pork chop	3 ounces	204	24	11	0	0	49
Prime rib	3 ounces	214	13	16	1	0	169
Ribs (pork)	3 ounces	185	23	9	0	0	44
Steak, filet mignon	3 ounces	152	23	5	0	0	50
Steak, New York strip	3 ounces	146	25	4	0	0	53
Steak, sirloin	3 ounces	156	26	4	0	0	54
Turkey, ground, 93% lean	3 ounces	128	15	7	0	0	59
Turkey bacon, extra lean	1 piece	20	3	0	0	0	120

BEANS

Food	Amount	Calories	Protein (g)	Fat (g)	Carbs (g)	Fiber (g)	Sodium (mg)
Black beans	½ cup cooked (no salt)	113	7	0	20	7	1
Black-eyed peas	½ cup cooked (no salt)	80	2	0	17	4	3
Fava beans	½ cup cooked (no salt)	94	6	0	16	4	4
Garbanzo (chickpeas)	½ cup cooked (no salt)	134	7	2	22	6	5
Kidney beans	½ cup cooked (no salt)	112	7	0	20	5	1
Lentil beans	½ cup cooked (no salt)	115	9	0	20	8	2
Lima beans	½ cup cooked (no salt)	104	6	0	20	4	14
Mung beans	½ cup cooked (no salt)	106	7	0	19	7	2
Navy beans	½ cup cooked (no salt)	91	7	0	24	9	0
Pinto beans	½ cup cooked (no salt)	122	7	0	22	7	1
Split peas	½ cup cooked (no salt)	116	8	0	20	8	2
Soybeans (edamame)	½ cup cooked (no salt)	94	8	4	8	4	4
Veggie patty	1 patty	138	18	4	7	6	411

DAIRY

Food	Amount	Calories	Protein (g)	Fat (g)	Carbs (g)	Fiber (g)	Sodium (mg)
Butter (salted)	1 tbsp.	100	0	11	0	0	81
Cheddar cheese	1 ounce	114	7	9	0	0	176
Cottage cheese (2%)	½ cup	102	15	2	4	0	459
Cottage cheese (1%)	½ cup	81	14	1	3	0	459
Egg	1 large	70	6	5	0	0	70
Goat cheese	1 ounce	75	5	6	0	0	103
Milk (2%)	1 cup	138	10	5	14	0	145
Milk (1%)	1 cup	102	8	2	13	0	107
Milk (skim)	1 cup	83	8	0	12	0	103
Mozzarella cheese	1 ounce	71	7	4	1	0	173
Muenster cheese	1 ounce	103	7	8	0	0	176
Pepperjack cheese	1 ounce	101	6	8	0	0	284
Swiss cheese	1 ounce	106	8	8	2	0	54
Yogurt, Greek (plain, 0% fat)	1 container (6 oz.)	100	18	0	7	0	80
Yogurt, Greek (plain, 2% fat)	1 container (6 oz.)	130	17	3	7	0	70
Yogurt (low-fat plain)	1 cup (8 oz.)	154	12	4	17	0	171
Yogurt (fat-free plain)	1 cup (8 oz.)	137	14	0	18	0	189

FRUIT

Food	Amount	Calories	Protein (g)	Fat (g)	Carbs (g)	Fiber (g)	Sodium (mg)
Apple	1 medium	93	0	0	24	4	2
Apricots	1 fruit	17	0	0	4	1	0
Banana	1 medium (7 inch)	105	1	0	27	3	1
Blackberries	½ cup	31	1	0	7	4	0
Blueberries	½ cup	42	0	0	10	2	0
Cantaloupe	1 cup (cubed)	54	0	0	7	1	0
Cherries	1 cup (w/ pits)	87	1	0	22	3	0
Clementine	1 fruit	35	1	0	9	1	1
Dates	1 date	20	0	0	5	1	0
Figs	1 medium	37	0	0	10	1	1
Grapefruit	½ medium	52	1	0	13	2	0
Grapes	1 cup (red or green seedless)	104	1	0	27	1	3
Guava	1 fruit	37	1	1	8	3	1
Honeydew	1 cup (cubed)	61	1	0	15	1	31
Kiwi	1 medium	46	1	0	11	2	2
Lemon	1 fruit	22	1	0	12	5	3
Lime	1 fruit	20	0	0	7	2	1
Mandarin	1 medium	47	1	0	12	2	2
Mango	½ cup (cubed)	53	1	0	14	1	1
Nectarine	1 medium	62	2	0	15	2	0
Orange	1 medium	65	1	0	16	3	0
Papaya	1 cup (cubed)	55	1	0	14	3	4
Peach	1 medium	59	1	0	15	2	0
Pear	1 medium	103	1	0	28	6	2
Persimmon	1 medium	32	0	0	8	2	0

Fruit, continued

Food	Amount	Calories	Protein (g)	Fat (g)	Carbs (g)	Fiber (g)	Sodium (mg)
Pineapple	1 slice	28	0	0	7	1	1
Plums	1 fruit	80	0	0	8	1	0
Pomegranate	½ cup (seeds)	72	1	1	16	3	3
Prunes	1 prune	23	0	0	6	1	0
Raisins, seedless	1 small box	129	1	0	34	2	5
Raspberries	1 cup	64	1	1	15	8	1
Strawberries	1 cup sliced	53	1	0	13	3	2
Tangerine	1 medium	47	1	0	12	2	2
Tomato	1 medium	22	1	0	5	1	6
Watermelon	1 wedge	86	2	0	22	1	3

VEGETABLES

Food	Amount	Calories	Protein (g)	Fat (g)	Carbs (g)	Fiber (g)	Sodium (mg)
Alfalfa sprouts	1 cup	8	1	0	1	1	2
Artichoke	1 medium	64	3	0	14	10	72
Arugula	½ cup	2	0	0	0	0	0
Asparagus	10 spears	30	3	0	6	3	3
Avocado	½ avocado	114	1	10	6	4	5
Bamboo shoots	½ cup raw	7	1	0	1	1	2
Beet greens	½ cup cooked	19	2	0	4	2	174
Beets	1 beet	35	1	0	8	2	64
Bell peppers	1 raw medium	24	1	0	6	2	4
Bok choy	½ cup cooked	10	1	0	1	1	29
Broccoli	½ cup cooked	15	1	0	3	1	15
Broccoli, raw	1 stalk	32	3	0	6	2	31
Brussels sprouts	½ cup cooked	28	2	0	6	2	16

Vegetables, continued

Food	Amount	Calories	Protein (g)	Fat (g)	Carbs (g)	Fiber (g)	Sodium (mg)
Cabbage	1 cup raw	17	1	0	4	1	13
Carrots	½ cup sliced	25	1	0	5	1	42
Cauliflower, raw	3 flowerets	10	0	0	2	1	12
Celery, raw	1 stalk	2	0	0	0	0	14
Chard	½ cup cooked (no salt)	18	1	0	3	1	157
Chives	1 tbsp. chopped	1	0	0	0	0	0
Collard greens	½ cup cooked (no salt)	25	2	0	4	2	15
Corn	1 medium ear	77	3	1	17	2	13
Cucumbers	½ cup sliced	8	0	0	1	0	1
Eggplant	½ cup cooked	17	0	0	4	1	0
Endive	½ cup chopped	4	0	0	1	1	5
Fennel	½ cup sliced	13	0	0	3	1	22
Garlic	1 clove	4	0	0	1	0	1
Green beans	½ cup cooked (no salt)	22	1	0	5	2	0
Green onions	1 stalk	3	0	0	1	0	0
Kale	1 cup raw	33	2	0	7	1	29
Leeks	1 leek	38	1	0	9	1	12
Lemon grass	1 cup raw	66	1	0	17	2	4
Lettuce, iceburg	½ cup	4	0	0	1	0	3
Lettuce, romaine	½ cup	5	0	0	0	0	0
Mushrooms	½ cup raw sliced	8	1	0	1	0	2
Mustard greens	½ cup cooked (no salt)	11	1	0	1	1	11
Okra	½ cup cooked (no salt)	18	1	0	4	2	5

Vegetables, continued

Food	Amount	Calories	Protein (g)	Fat (g)	Carbs (g)	Fiber (g)	Sodium (mg)
Olives, black	5 olives	15	0	2	0	0	130
Olives, green, Spanish w/ pimento	5 olives	25	0	2	1	0	240
Olive oil, extra virgin	1 tbsp.	120	0	14	0	0	0
Onion, raw	½ cup chopped	34	0	0	8	1	2
Parsley	½ cup chopped	11	0	0	1	1	17
Parsnip, raw	½ cup sliced	50	0	0	12	3	7
Peas	½ cup cooked	62	4	0	11	4	58
Potato, white	1 small with skin	60	1	0	13	2	24
Pumpkin	½ cup cooked	25	0	0	6	1	1
Radishes	1 medium	1	0	0	0	0	2
Radicchio	1 medium leaf	2	0	0	0	0	2
Rhubarb	1 stalk	11	0	0	2	0	2
Rutabaga	½ cup cooked	33	1	0	7	1	17
Sauerkraut	½ cup cooked (low sodium)	16	0	0	3	1	219
Spinach	½ cup cooked (no salt)	21	2	0	3	2	63
Spinach	1 cup raw	7	0	0	1	0	24
Summer squash	½ cup cooked	18	0	0	3	1	0
Sweet potato	1 small baked with skin	60	1	0	13	2	24
Swiss chard	½ cup cooked (no salt)	18	1	0	3	1	157
Turnip greens	½ cup cooked (no salt)	14	0	0	3	2	21
Turnips	1 small raw	19	0	0	4	1	46
Water chestnuts	½ cup raw	60	0	0	14	1	9

Vegetables, continued

Food	Amount	Calories	Protein (g)	Fat (g)	Carbs (g)	Fiber (g)	Sodium (mg)
Winter squash (Butternut)	½ cup cooked	41	0	0	10	1	4
Yam	1 cup cubed	158	2	0	37	5	11
Zucchini	½ cup sliced raw	10	0	0	2	0	5

NUTS AND SEEDS

Food	Amount	Calories	Protein (g)	Fat (g)	Carbs (g)	Fiber (g)	Sodium (mg)
Almonds, unsalted	20 almonds	139	5	12	4	2	0
Almond butter, unsalted	1 tbsp.	101	2	9	3	0	2
Brazil nuts	5 pieces	164	3	16	3	1	1
Cashews, unsalted	18 pieces	157	5	12	8	0	3
Cashew butter, unsalted	1 tbsp.	94	2	7	4	0	2
Peanuts, dry roasted, unsalted	20 pieces	117	4	9	4	1	1
Peanut butter, smooth, unsalted	1 tbsp.	94	4	8	3	1	2
Pecans, unsalted	19 halves	195	3	20	4	3	0
Pistachios, shelled	20 pieces	80	3	6	3	1	57
Pumpkin seeds, roasted, unsalted	42 pieces	63	2	2	7	1	2
Sesame seeds	1 tbsp.	51	1	4	2	1	1
Sunflower seeds, unsalted	¼ cup	186	6	15	7	3	1
Tahini	1 tbsp.	89	2	8	3	0	5
Walnuts, unsalted	14 halves	185	4	18	3	1	1

GRAINS

Food	Amount	Calories	Protein (g)	Fat (g)	Carbs (g)	Fiber (g)	Sodium (mg)
Bran flakes cereal	1 cup (without milk)	128	3	0	32	7	293
Brown rice pasta	1 ounce	106	2	1	22	1	3
Corn tortilla	1 tortilla	40	1	0	8	1	5
Oatmeal	½ cup dry oats	153	5	2	27	4	2
Pita, whole wheat	1 small	74	2	0	15	2	149
Popcorn, air popped, white, no salt	1 cup	31	1	0	6	1	0
Pumpernickel bread	1 slice	65	0	2	12	1	174
Quinoa, cooked, no salt	½ cup	111	4	1	19	2	6
Rice, brown, cooked, no salt	½ cup	108	2	0	22	1	5
Rice, white, cooked, no salt	½ cup	103	2	0	22	0	1
Rice, wild, cooked, no salt	½ cup	83	3	0	17	1	2
Rye bread	1 slice	83	2	1	15	1	211
Sourdough bread	1 slice	92	3	0	18	0	208
Sprouted bread	1 slice	80	4	0	15	3	75
Whole wheat bread	1 slice	100	3	0	22	2	410
Whole wheat pasta	1 cup cooked	176	7	0	37	4	4

Sources: www.nutritiondata.self.com and www.calorieking.com

APPENDIX II

Mix-and-Match Meal Plan

Here are seven examples for each mealtime that are simple and easy to make. Mix and match any breakfast, lunch, dinner, and snacks throughout the day. In total, there are forty-two options here to choose from! Vary the combinations or come up with your own healthy options for the full ten weeks. There is also a bonus (and optional) dessert section at the end.

BREAKFAST

1. 1 serving plain oatmeal (optional—add cinnamon, honey, berries, sliced banana, or any fruit of your choice)

   -or-

2. 2 free-range organic eggs with 1 piece gluten-free or whole grain toast and a small pat of real butter or 1 tsp. coconut spread (optional—make an omelet with eggs or egg whites, bell peppers, onions, mushrooms, or any of your favorite vegetables. Another option—add 1–2 pieces of low-sodium nitrate-free turkey bacon)

   -or-

3. 1 serving high-fiber cereal (at least 10 g fiber) with unsweetened almond milk, cashew milk, coconut milk, or organic milk (optional—add berries or 1 tsp. raw honey for sweetness)

   -or-

4. 1 slice gluten-free or whole grain toast with organic peanut butter or almond butter (optional—add spreadable raw honey)

-or-

5. 1 serving plain Greek yogurt with berries (optional—add chia seeds or sliced almonds for a little texture)

-or-

6. Fruit smoothie—½ to 1 cup plain Greek yogurt or unsweetened almond milk, then add your choice of fruit—½ banana, 1 cup fresh or frozen blueberries, strawberries, raspberries, blackberries, peaches, apricots, pineapple, etc. To add extra sweetness, add a little raw honey or stevia. Blend and enjoy.

-or-

7. Peanut butter, chocolate, and banana protein smoothie—1 cup ice, ½ cup unsweetened almond milk, 1 scoop chocolate whey or egg-white protein powder (make sure there are no artificial sweeteners or sucralose), 1 tbsp. organic peanut butter or almond butter, and ½ banana. Blend and enjoy.

MID-MORNING SNACK

1. 1 sliced apple with 1 tbsp. organic peanut butter or almond butter (optional—20 raw almonds or cashews instead of nut butter)

   -or-

2. 1 serving plain Greek yogurt with berries

   -or-

3. 1 natural/organic protein bar

   -or-

4. 1 slice gluten-free or whole-grain toast with organic peanut butter or almond butter

-or-

5. 2 hard-boiled organic eggs

   -or-

6. 20 unsalted almonds (or other nut of your choice)

   -or-

7. ½ avocado

LUNCH

1. Sandwich—2 slices gluten-free or whole grain toast, 2–3 slices organic, nitrate- and preservative-free lunch meat (turkey, chicken, ham, roast beef, etc.), lettuce or spinach, tomato, and mustard

   -or-

2. Grilled/baked organic chicken with ½ sweet potato and a small salad (optional—use any other protein you like instead of chicken)

   -or-

3. Mixed green or spinach salad with protein—Mix your favorite greens such as romaine lettuce, spinach, bell peppers, carrots, cucumbers, avocados, black olives, zucchini, onions, or tomatoes. Use chicken, salmon, steak, turkey, hard-boiled eggs, or beans as the protein. Mix 1–2 tbsp. olive oil and balsamic vinegar together as the dressing (optional—make a kale salad. Massage the leaves of the kale first with your hands to soften them. Then add the other ingredients)

   -or-

4. Leftovers from last night's dinner

   -or-

5. Homemade egg or chicken salad with rice crackers, in a wrap, or on a salad (be sure to go light on the mayo, or use mustard). Substitute plain Greek yogurt for the mayo to make this dish even healthier.

-or-

6. Salmon salad sandwich (can also be served on a salad or on lettuce leaves instead of bread)—Use 1 can of sockeye salmon or wild Alaskan salmon. A great substitute for tuna salad.

-or-

7. Organic turkey burger patty or hamburger patty served on lettuce (instead of a bun) with steamed vegetables

MID-AFTERNOON SNACK

1. 1 string cheese

   -or-

2. 2–4 slices of nitrate-free low-sodium or no-salt turkey wrapped around sliced red bell pepper (optional—dip in hummus)

   -or-

3. ½–1 cup blueberries, raspberries, blackberries, or cherries (optional—½ cup pomegranate seeds when in season)

   -or-

4. 1–2 tbsp. goat cheese on rice crackers

   -or-

5. Baby carrots, sliced bell peppers, and/or celery with hummus

   -or-

6. 20 unsalted almonds or other nuts

   -or-

7. ¼–⅓ cup homemade guacamole with 5–10 organic tortilla chips

DINNER

1. 3–4 oz. wild-caught or sockeye salmon with spinach or asparagus

   -or-

2. 3–4 oz. grilled organic chicken with steamed veggies

   -or-

3. 3–4 oz. grass-fed beef steak with broiled or grilled asparagus (optional—use any dark greens like spinach, Swiss chard, broccoli, mustard greens, broccolini, bok choy, etc.)

   -or-

4. 1 cup beans with ½ cup brown rice and a salad

   -or-

5. 4–5 medium turkey or grass-fed beef meatballs with low-sodium tomato sauce and a side salad (optional—use ground bison for the meatballs)

   -or-

6. 3–4 oz. tilapia with ½–1 cup quinoa and steamed zucchini (optional—use trout, cod, catfish, or halibut)

   -or-

7. 5–6 scallops with steamed spinach, Swiss chard, green beans, or asparagus (optional—use crab, lobster, or 5–6 grilled shrimp instead of scallops)

Note: The idea with the dinner options suggested here is to have a protein with vegetables—keep the carb content low. If you use a starch, keep the serving size small (e.g., ½ cup brown rice, ½ cup quinoa, ½ sweet potato, ½ plain baked potato, etc.).

Include many colorful veggies with your dinner. All the vegetable selections mentioned can be substituted with your favorites—peas, broccoli, Swiss chard, collard greens, bok choy, zucchini, asparagus, green beans, bell peppers, onions, etc. Likewise, all the protein selections mentioned can be swapped for your favorites.

DESSERT (OPTIONAL)

1. 1 tbsp. (about 10) dark chocolate chips (my first favorite!)

   -or-

2. 1–2 squares of dark chocolate—aim for 60 percent cacao or more (my second favorite!)

   -or-

3. 2–3 slices of watermelon or cantaloupe

   -or-

4. ½–1 cup strawberries or blueberries

   -or-

5. 5–10 frozen grapes

   -or-

6. ½–1 cup unsweetened chocolate almond milk

   -or-

7. ½–1 cup unsweetened apple sauce (add cinnamon if desired)

INDEX

ABOUT THE AUTHOR

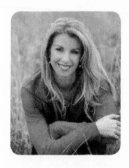

Justine SanFilippo graduated from the University of Notre Dame with a bachelor's degree in business administration. Since college (and since putting on 45 pounds while there!) she found her passion in health, wellness, and nutrition. She attended the Institute for Integrative Nutrition® in New York City in 2005 and became a certified health coach. There she received training from teachers such as Dr. Andrew Weil, Deepak Chopra, Dr. Mark Hyman, and David Wolfe. She is a certified personal trainer through the American Council on Exercise (ACE) and former owner of a gym. She also has a master's degree in human nutrition. Justine loves to teach others about health, wellness, fitness, and nutrition and help them reach their weight-loss goals.

Lose Your Inches without Losing Your Mind! is a down-to-earth and practical guide to lose inches in a healthy, balanced way without going completely bonkers! She started writing this book several years ago, purely out of the frustration of having tried every diet out there and being utterly confused along the way. After hitting many roadblocks, she finally found a simple solution to lose inches and keep them off that she wants to share with the world. Instead of confusing schedules and complicated strategies, she breaks her plan down into ten simple weeks so that people can achieve a smaller waistline while learning sustainable, healthy lifestyle habits.

Justine SanFilippo was also one of twenty-five experts who contributed to the Amazon bestseller *The Wellness Code—Your Ultimate Guide to Health, Fitness and Nutrition.*

Justine will eventually publish a children's book series as well. This series will teach children (and their parents) about making healthy choices in a fun and memorable way. There are many instances of childhood obesity that she thinks could be prevented. She hopes to make a difference by educating both the children and their parents in a simple, easy to understand way.

She looks forward to continuing to educate as many people as possible through her books, articles, seminars, workshops and speaking engagements. Her ultimate goal is to help millions of people be HAPPY, HEALTHY PEOPLE!

Please visit Justine online at www.happyhealthypeople.com

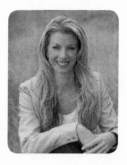

THANK YOU FOR PICKING UP THIS BOOK!

Get your FREE BONUSES to help you *Lose Your Inches* at
www.happyhealthypeople.com

Enter the secret code:
loseinchesnow

Want more help to lose your inches?
Go to www.happyhealthypeople.com for articles, products,
training programs and free videos.

Sample topics include:

How to slim your waistline without going bonkers

How to naturally boost your metabolism

How to lose belly fat

How often to eat throughout the day

How to break free from sugar cravings

How to reduce bloating

How to use coconut oil

How to fit exercise into your busy life

Going gluten free—is it right for me?

And much, much more!

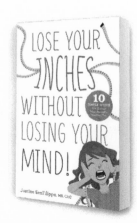

37993874R00120

Made in the USA
Charleston, SC
27 January 2015